EFFECTIVE PAIN MANAGEMENT

Fifth Edition

By

Rita Tamerius, RN, MN, NP

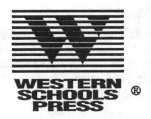

WESTERN
SCHOOLS ®
PRESS

21 Bristol Drive
South Easton, MA 02375
1-800-618-1670

ABOUT THE AUTHOR

Rita Tamerius, RN, MN, NP, coordinated the Multidiciplinary Pain Management Team for Green Hospital of Scripps Clinic in La Jolla, California. She was a faculty member at the University of Washington's School of Nursing, and has presented many seminars on the control of chronic pain and the role of the nurse caring for patients with cancer. She has written articles for the *California Nursing Review* and is currently consulting and lecturing in San Diego, California.

ABOUT THE REVIEWER

Mary E. A. Laskin, MN, RN, CS, has more than 12 years of experience in nursing, 7 of them in advanced practice roles. She has practiced as a clinical nurse specialist for medical-surgical nursing and pain management at Mercy Healthcare San Diego and acted as a pain consultant at LAC & USC Medical Center in Los Angeles. She earned her master's degree at UCLA School of Nursing, with a focus on pain management. She has presented many seminars for the professional and lay public on pain control, including oncology pain, sickle cell pain, pain in patients with AIDS, and pain in children. She has published in the *Journal of Advanced Medical-Surgical Nursing.* She is currently on the faculty for the ADN program at Maric College of Medical Careers in San Diego and consults on pain management issues.

Cindy Jones, RN, MS, OCN, and **Gloria York, RN, MAEd,** reviewed previous editions of this book.

Bibliographic citations corrected by: Anne Fredenburg Dolan, MEd

Copy Editor: Barbara Halliburton, PhD

Typesetter: Gwen Nichols

ISBN 1-878025-62-7

Library of Congress Catalog Card Number 94-60262

Western Schools courses are designed to provide Nursing professionals with the Educational information they need to enhance their career development. The information provided within these course materials is the result of research and consultation with prominent Nursing and Medical authorities and is, to the best of our knowledge, current and accurate. However, the courses and course materials are provided with the understanding that Western Schools is not engaged in offering legal, nursing, medical, or other professional advice.

Western Schools courses and course materials are not meant to act as a substitute for seeking out professional advice or conducting individual research. When applying the information provided in the courses and course materials to individual circumstances, all recommendations must be considered in light of the uniqueness pertaining to each situation.

Western Schools course materials are intended solely for *your* use, and *not* for the benefit of providing advice or recommendations to third parties. Western Schools devoids itself of any responsibility for adverse consequences resulting from the failure to seek nursing, medical or other professional advice. Western Schools further devoids itself of any responsibility for updating or revising any programs or publications presented, published, distributed or sponsored by Western Schools unless otherwise agreed to as part of an individual purchase contract.

IMPORTANT: Read these instructions *BEFORE* proceeding!

Enclosed with your course book you will find the FasTrax® answer sheet. Use this form to answer all the final exam questions that appear in this course book. If you are completing more than one course, be sure to write your answers on the appropriate answer sheet. Full instructions and complete grading details are printed on the FasTrax instruction sheet, also enclosed with your order. Please review them before starting. *If you are mailing your answer sheet(s) to Western Schools, we recommend you make a copy as a backup.*

ABOUT THIS COURSE

A "Pretest" is provided with each course to test your current knowledge base regarding the subject matter contained within this course. Your "Final Exam" is a multiple choice examination. **You will find the exam questions at the end of each chapter.** Some smaller hour courses include the exam at the end of the book.

In the event the course has less than 100 questions, mark your answers to the questions in the course book and leave the remaining answer boxes on the FasTrax answer sheet blank. Use a **black pen** to fill in your answer sheet.

A PASSING SCORE

You must score 70% or better in order to pass this course and receive your Certificate of Completion. Should you fail to achieve the required score, we will send you an additional FasTrax answer sheet so that you may make a second attempt to pass the course. Western Schools will allow you three chances to pass the same course…*at no extra charge!* After three failed attempts to pass the same course, your file will be closed.

RECORDING YOUR HOURS

Please monitor the time it takes to complete this course using the handy log sheet on the other side of this page. See below for transferring study hours to the course evaluation.

COURSE EVALUATIONS

In this course book you will find a short evaluation about the course you are soon to complete. This information is vital to providing the school with feedback on this course. The course evaluation answer section is in the lower right hand corner of the FasTrax answer sheet marked "Evaluation" with answers marked 1–25. Your answers are important to us, please take five minutes to complete the evaluation.

On the back of the FasTrax instruction sheet there is additional space to make any comments about the course, the school, and suggested new curriculum. Please mail the FasTrax instruction sheet, with your comments, back to Western Schools in the envelope provided with your course order.

TRANSFERRING STUDY TIME

Upon completion of the course, transfer the total study time from your log sheet to question #25 in the Course Evaluation. The answers will be in ranges, please choose the proper hour range that best represents your study time. You MUST log your study time under question #25 on the course evaluation.

EXTENSIONS

You have 2 years from the date of enrollment to complete this course. A six (6) month extension may be purchased. If after 30 months from the original enrollment date you do not complete the course, *your file will be closed and no certificate can be issued.*

CHANGE OF ADDRESS?

In the event you have moved during the completion of this course please call our student services department at 1-800-618-1670 and we will update your file.

A GUARANTEE YOU'LL GIVE HIGH HONORS TO

If any continuing education course fails to meet your expectations or if you are not satisfied in any manner, for any reason, you may return it for an exchange or a refund (less shipping and handling) within 30 days. Software, video and audio courses must be returned unopened.

Thank you for enrolling at Western Schools!

WESTERN SCHOOLS
P.O. Box 1930
Brockton, MA 02303
(800) 618-1670

EFFECTIVE PAIN MANAGEMENT

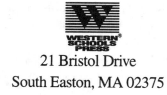

21 Bristol Drive
South Easton, MA 02375

Please use this log to total the number of hours you spend reading the text and taking the final examination (use 50-min hours).

Date	Hours Spent
_____	_____
_____	_____
_____	_____
_____	_____
_____	_____
_____	_____
_____	_____
_____	_____
_____	_____
_____	_____
_____	_____
_____	_____
_____	_____

TOTAL [ ]

Please log your study hours with submission of your final exam. To log your study time, fill in the appropriate circle under question 25 of the FasTrax® answer sheet under the "Evaluation" section.

PLEASE LOG YOUR STUDY HOURS WITH SUBMISSION OF YOUR FINAL EXAM. Please choose which best represents the total study hours it took to complete this 30 hour course.

A. less than 25 hours

B. 25–28 hours

C. 29–32 hours

D. greater than 32 hours

EFFECTIVE PAIN MANAGEMENT

WESTERN SCHOOLS' NURSING
CONTINUING EDUCATION EVALUATION

Instructions: Mark your answers to the following questions with a black pen on the "Evaluation" section of your FasTrax® answer sheet provided with this course. You should not return this sheet. Please use the scale below to rate the following statements:

A Agree Strongly   **C Disagree Somewhat**
B Agree Somewhat   **D Disagree Strongly**

The course content met the following education objectives:

1. Recognized the purpose of pain and how pain is described and classified.

2. Recognized cognitive and social factors that affect the experience of pain.

3. Discussed the two major models of pain and the processes involved in pain conduction.

4. Recognized components, tools, and guidelines for physical assessment of patients with pain and the attitudes that patients and health-care professionals may have toward pain.

5. Discussed guidelines and techniques used to relieve pain and their various advantages and disadvantages.

6. Described the mechanisms, durations, onsets and major side effects of analgesics and specified dosages equianalgesic to morphine.

7. Discussed the drugs used for moderate to severe pain, the advantages and disadvantages of their use, and their major side effects.

8. Stated the prevalence of postoperative pain, descriptions used for pain, and the results of inadequate and adequate pain treatment.

9. Described special pain problems in children, specified approaches used in treatment, and results of studies on pain in this age group.

10. Recognized mechanisms, signs, symptoms, and treatments of headaches, phantom limb pain, and trigeminal neuralgia.

11. Recognized sources, severity, management techniques, and treatment of pain associated with cancer.

12. Described types of chronic pain disorders and the problems related to these disorders.

13. Described special pain problems of the elderly, key assessment techniques, and specified approaches used in treatment.

14. The content of this course was relevant to the objectives.

15. This offering met my professional education needs.

16. The objectives met the overall purpose/goal of the course.

17. The course was generally well written and the subject matter explained thoroughly? (If no please explain on the back of the FasTrax instruction sheet.)

18. The content of this course was appropriate for home study.

19. The final examination was well written and at an appropriate level for the content of the course.

Please complete the following research questions in order to help us better meet your educational needs. Pick the ONE answer which is most appropriate.

20. What nursing shift do you most commonly work?

    A. Morning Shift (Any shift starting after 3:00am or before 11:00am)

    B. Day/Afternoon Shift (Any shift starting after 11:00am or before 7:00pm)

    C. Night Shift (Any shift starting after 7:00pm or before 3:00am)

    D. I work rotating shifts

21. What was the SINGLE most important reason you chose this course?

    A. Low Price

    B. New or Newly revised course

    C. High interest/Required course topic

    D. Number of Contact Hours Needed

22. Where do you work? (If your place of employment is not listed below, please leave this question blank.)

    A. Hospital

    B. Medical Clinic/Group Practice/ HMO/Office setting

    C. Long Term Care/Rehabilitation Facility/Nursing Home

    D. Home Health Care Agency

23. Which field do you specialize in?

    A. Medical/Surgical

    B. Geriatrics

    C. Pediatrics/Neonatal

    D. Other

24. For your last renewal, how many months BEFORE your license expiration date did you order your course materials?

    A. 1–3 months

    B. 4–6 months

    C. 7–12 months

    D. Greater than 12 months

25. **PLEASE LOG YOUR STUDY HOURS WITH SUBMISSION OF YOUR FINAL EXAM.** Please choose which best represents the total study hours it took to complete this 30 hour course.

    A. less than 25 hours

    B. 25–28 hours

    C. 29–32 hours

    D. greater than 32 hours

CONTENTS

Effective Pain Management

PRETEST

Begin by taking the pretest. Compare your answers on the pretest to the answer key (located in the back of the book). Circle those test items that you missed. The pretest answer key indicates the course chapters where the content of that question is discussed.

Next, read each chapter. Focus special attention on the chapters where you made incorrect answer choices. Study questions are provided at the end of each chapter so you can assess your progress and understanding of the material.

The answer choices to the following questions are:

a. True   b. False

1. The average adult loses about 23 days each year because of pain-related problems.

2. Pain can be defined as a syndrome of behavioral and physical manifestations that can be objectively detected by the nurse.

3. Anxiety plays a key role in the cognitive perception of pain.

4. The gate control theory of pain proposed that pain could be relieved by altering a person's thought processes.

5. The intensity of pain should be rated by the nurse, not the patient.

6. Patients should be encouraged to wait until their pain is more than mild before requesting pain medication.

7. Relaxation techniques can reduce pain by reducing stress and muscle tension, which play a key role in prolonging pain.

8. Nonopioid analgesics act peripherally, by preventing synthesis of prostaglandins.

9. One hundred milligrams of meperidine given intramuscularly is equal to 10 mg of morphine given by the same route.

10. The earliest indication that tolerance is developing to an opioid is the patient's complaint that the duration of the drug's effectiveness is decreased.

INTRODUCTION

No medical problem or stress is more widespread than pain. The prevalence of both chronic and acute pain is staggering. In addition, as the average age of the population increases over the next decades, the number of persons who have pain is certain to increase dramatically.

THE SCOPE OF THE PROBLEM

One of the most common problems, lower back pain, accounts for more than 8 million visits to physicians' offices each year and has disabled an estimated 7 million Americans (Donovan & Girton, 1984). According to the American Migraine Study, 18% of females and 6% of males in the United States currently have severe migraine headaches (Lipton & Stewart, 1993). An estimated 20 million to 50 million Americans have arthritic pain.

In a 1985 study, 21 million adults (13%) reported experiencing chronic pain for at least 101 days in the preceding year. All persons with pain stated that it lowered the quality of their lives by interfering with daily routines, making it difficult to concentrate on their work, and preventing them from fully enjoying their leisure time and activities (Sternbach, 1987).

The economic consequences of chronic and acute pain are also startling. The estimated annual cost of lower back pain alone is more than $50 billion, possibly as high as $100 billion (Frymoyer & Cats-Baril, 1991). The avenge adult loses about 23 days each year because of pain. The average full-time worker loses 5 working days each year. Nationwide, this adds up to 550 million days in a single year.

Undertreatment of pain is such a significant problem that acute pain was one of the first clinical conditions for which the Agency for Health Care Policy and Research (AHCPR) developed treatment guidelines. An interdisciplinary panel did an extensive literature search and, when possible, used meta-analysis to evaluate the data. They also obtained opinions from external consultants and received testimony at an open forum. The guidelines received major media attention when they were published in February 1992. They include a pamphlet for patients that is designed to be completed with the help of the patients' doctors and nurses. AHCPR is currently developing guidelines for treatment of pain due to cancer.

It is not surprising then that health care professionals spend much of their time dealing with pain and pain-related problems. Nurses, no matter what their clinical specialties, are expected to have special knowledge about how to relieve pain. Even those who spend their day in neonatal intensive care, an operating room, or at home taking care of young children find that their families, next-door neighbors, and acquaintances expect them to know more than the general public about relieving pain.

The purpose of this text is to provide information that will make you more effective in relieving pain. Because nurses are usually the health team members in the best position to ascertain the need for pain relief and to select the most appropriate measures to relieve pain, major emphasis is placed on what nurses can do to improve pain relief. The structure used is the nursing process: assessing and diagnosing the patient's pain, developing a plan for interventions, and then evaluating that plan. Sometimes the interventions can be initiated without a physician's order. However, because most of the interventions used to relieve severe pain are directed by physicians, many of the suggestions are targeted to help nurses improve the effectiveness of the medical treatments for pain.

This book examines the pain phenomenon, including variability, causes, and ways to alleviate it. Readers will learn what is known about the physiological and psychological bases of pain. The misconceptions of patients and health care professionals that interfere with pain relief are also discussed.

Finally, special emphasis is given to the proper uses of analgesics. Nurses, more than any other health team member, are in the best position to select the proper routes and doses of analgesics for their patients. This requires an in-depth understanding of the indications, contraindications, side effects, and potency of these medications.

The subject of pain and pain control is complex and vast. Therefore, this book gives priority to information that directly contributes to nurses' understanding of likely situations and the types of interventions over which nurses most likely have some control. Many theoretical considerations and research are summarized only briefly. The Bibliography lists extensive references to which students can turn for in-depth information.

This book is not intended to prepare nurses to work as specialists in pain control or in specialized pain control centers. It is designed to meet the information needs of nurses who work in a wide variety of settings and those who are temporarily retired.

OVERALL LEARNING OBJECTIVE

Pain problems are ubiquitous. The purpose of this course is to prepare nurses to better deal with pain problems by increasing their understanding of the basic pathophysiology and psychology of pain, the variety of problems associated with pain, the proper uses of pain relief interventions, and the role of the nurse in pain management. The textbook itself is intended to serve as an ongoing reference for nurses as they encounter pain-related problems at home and in the workplace.

CHAPTER 1

THE PUZZLE OF PAIN

CHAPTER OBJECTIVE

After studying this chapter, the reader will be able to recognize the purpose of pain and how pain is described and classified.

LEARNING OBJECTIVES

After studying this chapter, the reader will be able to

1. Indicate the purpose the ability to feel pain plays in protecting a person's health.

2. Recognize examples of two of the five different types of pain.

3. Specify two of the major classes of terms used to describe the qualities of pain.

INTRODUCTION

Pain is a nearly universal experience and has been the subject of intense speculation and treatment for centuries. However, no one has ever been able to define it satisfactorily. It is so variable and it occurs in such a diversity of situations that no single definition is adequate. All experts agree, however, that pain is unpleasant and a complex phenomenon.

This book uses the following two definitions. The first is Margo McCaffery's operational definition: "Pain is whatever the experiencing person says it is, existing whenever he says it does" (McCaffery, 1979). The second is the one adopted by the International Association for the Study of Pain (IASP) and the Oncology Nursing Society: "Pain is an unpleasant sensory and emotional experience associated with actual or potential tissue damage or described in terms of such damage" (Merskey, 1979). Both definitions address the emotional and subjective dimension of pain, as well as its sensory dimension.

THE BENEFITS OF PAIN

Everyone has occasionally wished that he or she could be impervious to pain. Most persons, however, recognize that pain plays an essential role in protecting their health. Pain has three main purposes:

1. To warn us before serious injury takes place. For example, when we touch a hot stove or other potentially damaging object, pain causes us to withdraw before we are injured. Another example is the abdominal pain that occurs before the impending rupture of an

inflamed appendix, thus allowing sufficient time for surgical intervention to prevent potentially lethal peritonitis.

2. To teach us to avoid dangerous objects or situations. For instance, children usually require only one experience with a hot stove to learn that they should avoid stoves.

3. To prevent further injury to an injured region of the body. The pain produced by a damaged organ, joint, or other tissues forces us to protect that area from further injury by limiting our activities until recovery is well under way.

The significant benefits of being able to feel pain can be appreciated by studying those rare individuals who have a congenital inability to feel it. The best documented case is a Miss C. She was a student at McGill University when she first came to the attention of physicians in the Montreal area. Her father, a physician, was fully aware of her problems.

Miss C. was highly intelligent and appeared normal in every way except that she had never felt pain. Because of this abnormality, when she was a child, she bit off the tip of her tongue while chewing food and sustained a third-degree burn when she knelt on a radiator to look out a window. The physicians in Montreal were astonished to learn that she could not remember ever having sneezed or coughed and to find that she had virtually no gag and corneal reflexes. Before she was 20 years old, Miss C. already had severe health problems because of her insensitivity to pain.

Because she did not turn over during sleep, shift her weight when standing for long periods, or protect vulnerable joints from overextension, Miss C. had severe inflammation of her knees, hips, and spine. Her condition, called Charcot's joint, is seen in patients who have abnormal innervation of one or more joints. The greatest problems develop in those joints that are often injured slightly in everyday life: ankles, knees, wrists, and elbows.

Most persons who painfully overstretch a joint, such as the ankle, protect that joint from further trauma by favoring it. They put an elastic bandage around the ankle and limp or even use crutches to reduce weight-bearing until healing is well under way. Persons who have no or reduced pain sensations continue to use the joint normally, despite the injury. The repeated trauma to the ligaments and other tissues eventually results in severe inflammation and finally necrosis as the blood supply becomes diminished. The presence of dead and dying tissues in and around the joint capsule leads to the development of osteomyelitis in the nearby bones. Systemic bacterial infections begin to develop as a result of the joint disease. These can be controlled initially with drugs, but ultimately the organisms become resistant to even the most powerful antibiotics. Miss C. died at the age of 29 as a result of overwhelming septicemia.

PAIN WITHOUT INJURY

Because tissue damage and pain so often occur together, most persons assume that the two are invariably linked. Several definitions of pain, in fact, reinforce this misconception. For example, Mountcastle (1980) defines pain as the sensory experience evoked by stimuli that injure or threaten to destroy tissue. As intuitively attractive as this definition is, it is incorrect. Although pain and real or threatened tissue damage are often linked, the relationship is so variable that pain cannot be defined exclusively in terms of tissue damage.

A vivid example of a common situation in which pain is marked but tissue damage is minor is normal labor and delivery. After studying the level of pain reported by women undergoing prepared childbirth, Melzack concluded, "Labor is . . . among the most severe pains that have been recorded" (Melzack & Wall, 1983). Yet a normal birth produces relatively trivial damage to the mother's tissues, and the pain associated with it does not serve as a warning of potential injury. If pain is defined exclusively in terms of the potential or actual production of tissue damage, the sensations experienced during normal childbirth do not fit the definition.

Another case in which pain is severe despite the absence of ongoing or potential tissue damage is severe nerve injury, particularly injuries to the brachial plexus. This latter type of nerve injury occurs more often as the number of motorcycle accidents increases each year. The usual scenario is for a cyclist to hit an obstruction and be thrown forward over the bike's handlebars. Hitting the road at about the same speed the bike was traveling, the cyclist usually lands with arms extended in front. The impact wrenches the shoulders down and back. In the most severe cases, the brachial plexus in one or both shoulders is torn away (avulsed) from the spinal cord. No repair is possible.

Even though one or both arms are without sensation from the shoulder down, arm pain is a problem for many of these patients for months or years after the tissues are healed. Melzack and Wall (1983) described an Air Force pilot who had this syndrome:

> His right arm was completely paralyzed from the shoulder down. . . . The limp arm was totally anesthetic, so that he had no sensation of any stimuli applied to it. On being questioned, he stated that he could sense very clearly an entire arm, but it had no relationship to his real arm. This "phantom" arm seemed to him to be placed across his chest while the real paralyzed arm hung at his side. The phantom never moved and the fingers were tightly clenched in a cramped fist with the nails digging into the palm. The entire arm felt as though it was on fire.

Chronic pain after severe nerve injury is quite common. A 1980 study of 100 consecutive cases of avulsion of the brachial plexus showed that 95 of the 100 patients were in severe pain. Their descriptions of their phantoms and their pain were similar to those of the Air Force pilot.

SERIOUS INJURY WITHOUT PAIN

Studies of soldiers injured in battle provide further proof that no consistent link exists between tissue damage and pain. As many as 65% of severely wounded soldiers report little or no pain for hours or days after being injured. About 20% of patients undergoing major surgery have a similar absence of severe pain.

THE LANGUAGE OF PAIN

Unfortunately, no common language or terminology is used to discuss pain and pain-related problems. This leads to unnecessary difficulties in communication not only among professionals but also between clinicians and patients. The following sections cover the major terms used in this course and the manner in which they are used.

Categories of Pain

Pain is generally categorized into five different types:

1. Acute pain. This type of pain is usually self-limiting and lasts less than 6 months. The term *acute* refers only to the duration of the pain. It provides no information about the pain's intensity, source, or quality. The underlying cause of the pain is usually known. Everyone has experienced acute pain.

- Examples: headaches, postoperative pain, childbirth, injuries, sore throat, dental procedures

2. Chronic pain. This type of pain lasts 6 months or longer. The term *chronic* should not be construed to mean that the pain is not severe. Chronic pain covers the full spectrum of pain intensity.

3. Chronic periodic pain. This type of pain is intermittent. Episodes of pain occur at intervals over months and years. Although periods lasting for days or weeks may be pain-free, the pain eventually returns.

   - Examples: migraine headache, back pain, trigeminal neuralgia

4. Chronic benign pain. This type of pain is present most of the time, but its intensity varies. The term *benign* refers to the fact that the underlying cause of the pain is not life-threatening. It is often misinterpreted to mean that no physical abnormality is associated with the pain or that the pain is not a serious problem. This is unfortunate, because chronic pain is certainly not benign (Boas, 1976).

   - Examples: back or neck pain, arthritis, headaches

5. Chronic progressive pain. This type of pain is most commonly associated with malignant tumors. The underlying physical abnormality is usually known and is life-threatening.

Because the effects of moderate to severe pain lasting more than a month are similar to the effects of chronic pain, this textbook uses the term *prolonged pain* to refer to pain that lasts longer than a few weeks and significantly interferes with the patient's quality of life. Readers should be aware, however, that prolonged pain is not widely accepted as a separate classification for pain.

Descriptions of Pain

Anyone who has had severe pain who has attempted to describe it to a physician or friend knows that it is difficult to find words that really convey what the pain feels like. The reason for the loss for words is not that these words do not exist. Rather, it is because these are not terms that most persons use frequently. As Melzack and Wall (1983) accurately point out, "The words may seem absurd: . . . 'it feels as if someone is shoving a red-hot poker through my toes and slowly twisting it around.' " Yet these as-if statements often convey the unique qualities of the patient's pain better than any clinical terms can.

Significant strides have been made toward providing clinicians, patients, and researchers with a means of describing the qualities of pain. Four major classes of terms are required:

1. Sensory terms. Words that describe the sensory qualities of the experience in terms of time, space, pressure, temperature, and other properties (e.g., a bursting sensation, hot poker, drilling pressure).

2. Affective terms. Words that describe affective qualities, in terms of tension, fear, and autonomic responses that are part of the pain experience (e.g., makes me break into a cold sweat, patient's pulse and blood pressure increased).

3. Evaluative terms. Words that describe the subjective overall intensity of the total pain experience (e.g., unbearable, excruciating, tolerable).

4. Temporal terms. Words that describe pain in relationship to time patterns (e.g., occurs after I eat, present only in the morning).

Using this information, Melzack developed a pain questionnaire (Appendix A) that provides clinicians with greater insight into the qualities that make up the pain experience for different persons. Although no test can precisely describe a person's experience of pain, this tool does provide an improved means by which patients can communicate their painful sensations to others.

Usefulness of Pain Description in Diagnosis

Persons with the same types of painful conditions use the same types of words to describe the pain. Sometimes the words are so highly specific to the underlying abnormality that a diagnosis can almost be made without seeing the patient. For example, if a patient with an eye problem says his eye feels as if it has something irritating it, the physician will be less concerned than if the patient describes the discomfort as a dull ache or a sharp pain.

Table 1-1 lists descriptors frequently used by patients with one of eight different pain syndromes. Only words used by more than one third of the patients with each condition are listed. The numbers in parentheses are the actual percentages of patients who used each word (Melzack & Wall, 1983).

SUMMARY

Health care professionals should become thoroughly familiar with the language of pain and use it when assessing patients and documenting findings in the patients' medical records. Chapters 2 and 3 discuss the physiological and psychological factors that influence how intensely a person experiences a painful stimuli.

TABLE 1-1
Descriptive Terms Characteristic of Selected Pain Syndromes

Syndrome	Sensory	Affective	Evaluative	Temporal
Menstrual pain	Cramping (44) Aching (44)	Sickening (56) Tiring (44)		Constant (56)
Arthritic pain	Aching (50) Gnawing (38)	Exhausting (46)	Annoying (38)	Rhythmic (91) Constant (44)
Labor pain	Cramping (82) Sharp (64) Shooting (46) Aching (46) Stabbing (40) Pounding (37)	Exhausting (46) Tiring (36) Fearful (36)	Intense (46)	Rhythmic (91)
Disk disease pain	Sharp (60) Shooting (50) Tender (50) Throbbing (40) Cramping (40) Aching (40) Heavy (40) Stabbing (40)	Tiring (46) Exhausting (40)	Unbearable (40)	Rhythmic (70)
Cancer pain	Shooting (50) Sharp (50) Gnawing (50) Burning (50) Heavy (50)	Exhausting (50)	Unbearable (50)	Constant (100) Rhythmic (88)
Phantom limb pain	Stabbing (50) Cramping (50) Burning (50) Sharp (38) Throbbing (38) Aching (38)	Tiring (50) Exhausting (38) Cruel (38)		Constant (88) Rhythmic (63)
Postherpetic pain	Sharp (84) Pulling (67) Aching (50) Tender (83)	Exhausting (50)		Constant (50)

Note: Numbers in parentheses are percentage of patients who used the term.

Source: Melzck & Wall, 1983.

EXAM QUESTIONS

Chapter 1

Questions 1–5

1. Childbirth is an example of what type of pain?

   a. Chronic
   b. Acute, progressive
   c. Chronic benign
   d. Acute

2. Which of the four major classes of terms for describing pain contains words that describe the experience in terms of time, space, pressure, temperature, and other properties?

   a. Evaluative
   b. Sensory
   c. Affective
   d. Temporal

3. Mr. Jones has been having about six migraine headaches per year since he was 12 years old. In which of the following categories would his pain be classified?

   a. Chronic periodic pain
   b. Acute pain
   c. Chronic benign pain
   d. Acute periodic pain

4. Which of the four major classes of terms for describing pain contains words that describe the subjective overall intensity of the total pain experience?

   a. Evaluative
   b. Affective
   c. Sensory
   d. Temporal

5. Which of the following statements accurately describes one of the three main purposes pain serves in protecting a person's health?

   a. It teaches our bodies the type of damage taking place.
   b. It shows us that injury and pain always go together.
   c. It tells us the severity of the injury we have sustained.
   d. It warns us before serious injury takes place.

CHAPTER 2

HOW THE MIND AFFECTS THE PAIN EXPERIENCE

CHAPTER OBJECTIVE

After studying this chapter, the reader will be able to recognize cognitive and social factors that affect the experience of pain.

LEARNING OBJECTIVES

After studying this chapter, the reader will be able to

1. Select the correct definition for placebo.

2. Recognize one of the cognitive influences on the pain experience.

3. Specify one of the social influences on the pain experience.

4. Specify the number of patients in 10 that research has shown will respond favorably to placebos at one time or another.

INTRODUCTION

Differences in the ability and willingness to tolerate pain can be seen every day. Most are due to psychological rather than physiological factors. This does not mean that persons who experience greater pain are exaggerating or imagining their pain. Rather, psychological factors influence the transmission of painful stimuli to the central nervous system, and other cognitive factors influence how the stimuli are interpreted and acted on.

PAIN AND THE MIND

Long before any scientific understanding of the role the mind plays in the perception of pain, it was recognized that suffering could be reduced by certain "mind tricks." For example, folk medicine has long included numerous remedies that use techniques such as distraction, counterirritants, and suggestion to reduce a patient's pain experience. Only recently have scientists discovered the underlying mechanisms that make these remedies so effective.

The powerful influence of the mind became apparent as scientists began to study pain systematically. For instance, when heat was applied to the skin of test subjects, nearly all of them reported feeling the sensation of heat at approximately the same temperature, regardless of their age, sex, education, or racial or cultural backgrounds. However, the point at which the sensation became painful differed significantly from subject to subject. Experiments such as these suggest that the point, or threshold, at which persons can feel pressure, heat, or cold is similar for everyone. What differs is the point at which the sensation becomes painful. The many factors that account for these differences are discussed in the next section.

COGNITIVE INFLUENCES ON THE PERCEPTION OF PAIN

What a person thinks about a physical sensation has a tremendous impact on how the person reacts to it and ultimately determines whether the sensation is classified as pleasurable or painful. This occurs because sensations created by a painful (or any other) stimulus are not perceived until the cerebral cortex has acted on them.

Potential Meaning of the Pain

The potential implications of the pain being experienced affect how intensely the pain is felt. To illustrate this point, imagine that you have just noticed an aching sensation in your little finger. You probably would not pay much attention to this ache. Suppose, however, you felt a similar ache substernally. Suddenly the ache would seem more significant and painful. Why? The explanation is that the possible implications a painful sensation holds for an individual can greatly magnify or reduce the amount of

pain being experienced. An ache in a little finger is usually trivial, whereas a substernal ache might indicate a heart problem, a potentially life-threatening condition. Consequently, you become more anxious and focus more attention on the sensations when the pain is substernal.

Setting in Which Pain Occurs

The environment or situation in which a painful stimulus occurs also can greatly reduce or magnify how intensely the stimulus is felt. Using the example of the finger ache again, suppose the ache occurred while you were playing an exciting tennis game. Most likely you would ignore the ache or never even notice it in the first place. On the other hand, if the same ache occurred just as you were trying to fall asleep, you might find it difficult to ignore. Why? The lack of distractions in the environment would make the ache seem more intense and more difficult to ignore.

Anxiety Level

In physiological terms, anxiety is a state of apprehensiveness associated with physiological changes caused by stimulation of the sympathetic and parasympathetic nervous systems (i.e., tachycardia, sweating, increased blood pressure). A person's level of anxiety can notably influence the response to painful stimuli. Anxiety can lower the pain threshold, and it can cause additional painful stimuli (e.g., muscle spasm). A high level of anxiety can also make a person more susceptible to fears that the pain may be a symptom of some dire condition.

Much about the relationship between pain and anxiety is still unknown. Talbot et al. (1991) used positron emission tomography (PET) and magnetic resonance imaging (MRI) to examine the role of the cerebral cortex in pain. They found that noxious thermal stimulation activated the somatosensory cortex and a region of the limbic system called the anterior cingulate gyrus. This region is thought to control emotion, especially anxiety. The investigators proposed that although the sensory information about pain is processed in the somatosensory cortex, the emotional response is processed in the limbic region. The study shows that the association between pain and anxiety may have a physiological basis.

Perceived Control over Painful Stimuli

Studies have shown that persons have greater discomfort with pain they cannot control. On the other hand, if a person thinks that he or she can exert even a small degree of control over a painful stimulus, that person will suffer less distress. For example, when patients in a burn unit were allowed to participate in the debridement of their burned tissues, they claimed that the process was much more bearable than when they did not participate (Bond, 1984). Similarly, for women in childbirth, the severity of pain experienced during childbirth is perceived to be less when the women use special breathing and relaxation techniques to exert some control over their pain during labor and delivery.

The Power of Suggestion

Suggestion has a powerful effect on the perceived intensity of pain. The analgesic power of placebos is a good example of this. A placebo can be defined as any medical treatment or nursing care (medication or procedure, including surgery) that produces an effect in a patient that is due to the implicit or explicit therapeutic intent of the placebo and not to its specific nature (physical or chemical properties). A patient who responds to a placebo in accordance with its intent is a placebo reactor. The response is called a positive placebo response. Although not everyone is a responder, about 9 of 10 subjects will respond favorably to a placebo at one time or another (Houde, Wallenstein, & Rogers, 1960).

One study of the effectiveness of placebos found that severe pain could be relieved in approximately 35% of patients when a placebo was given in place of morphine or other analgesic. This is a remarkably high

degree of pain relief, inasmuch as large doses of morphine relieve pain in only about 75% of patients (Beecher, 1946).

Various mechanisms have been suggested to explain the placebo response. Two proposed mechanisms are anxiety reduction and classical conditioning. Reducing a person's anxiety could decrease pain by raising the person's threshold to pain and increasing muscle relaxation. Classical conditioning could reduce the perception of pain in persons who strongly believe that the pills or injections will provide pain relief, probably through conditioned physiological responses (e.g., increased secretion of endorphins).

Unfortunately, myths about placebo responses lead to unnecessary pain for some patients. McCaffery (1979) notes the following in her textbook on pain management for nurses:

> The most serious problem with placebos is that when a patient receives pain relief from a "sugar pill," some health team members will draw erroneous conclusions. Even if it is never openly spoken, it is clear that these team members view the patient as some sort of "neurotic" or a "stupid" individual whose pain does not originate with any physical or physiological stimulus. It is thought that the patient is either deliberately faking the pain or "just thinks he or she has pain."

> A true and positive placebo response absolutely cannot be used to diagnose pain as psychogenic rather than somatogenic. Likewise, it cannot be used to diagnose malingering.

> It is a gross injustice to the patient to believe that his positive placebo response means he is a stupid or neurotic person who has no cause to feel pain in the first place. A much more accurate conclusion about the placebo reactor is that he very much wants

to be relieved of his pain and that he trusts something or someone, perhaps the nurse, to help him obtain pain relief. I feel that misunderstanding such a patient is one of the saddest and most lamentable occurrences in all of health care.

The deliberate use of placebos is on the decline. This is fortunate, because most often placebos were ordered in a misguided and futile attempt to diagnose malingering. No matter what the patient's response, the usual outcome was increasing suspicion about the patient's pain on the part of the health team and a consequent decline in the patient's sense of trust. In addition to the placebo's uselessness as a means of detecting malingerers, moral, ethical, and legal issues must be considered when a sugar pill or a saline injection is given to an unsuspecting patient in place of an analgesic.

SOCIAL INFLUENCES ON THE PAIN EXPERIENCE

Childhood Experiences

In some families, children receive a tremendous amount of attention and sympathy for even the smallest bruise or cut. In other families, children are told not to cry when hurt. Injuries are downplayed or even ignored. These early childhood experiences with pain and how to cope with it have a lifelong impact on how each person reacts to painful stimuli.

Gender

Pain behaviors are generally more acceptable in women than men. Armitage, Schneiderman, and Bass (1979) found that physicians did much more thorough workups of male patients than of female patients with the same complaint. The researchers speculated that the physicians were responding to the stereotype that men are more stoic than women. McCaffery and Ferrell (1992) conducted a survey to determine nurses' perception of gender influences on pain. Although 63% noted that men and women have the same sensitivity to pain, 47% thought that women tolerate more pain than men do. Fifty-three percent thought that men tend to underreport pain, and 48% stated that women were more expressive. Note that these are the nurses' perceptions, not actual findings among persons in pain. The results suggest that nurses might have preconceptions about how their patients will respond to pain. Such preconceptions might affect assessment of patients.

Ethnic Background

Ethnic background or culture determines the way persons solve their problems and derive meaning from their lives. It teaches behaviors, including pain behaviors. Different cultures use different types of terms to describe pain (e.g., in emotional or physical terms). These differences should not be ignored. They also should not be used to prejudge a patient.

Many nurses do prejudge patients on the basis of cultural characteristics. In a study by Davitz and Davitz (1985), nurses reviewed vignettes about patients and rated the degree of physical pain and psychological distress they thought each patient would have. The only differences between patients were their ethnic and religious backgrounds. The results are indicated in the following as nurses' inferences.

- Asian. In many Asian cultures, it is considered disgraceful to cry or complain of pain, even during extremely painful procedures. Because of this, Asians may not expect to receive pain medication. Therefore, they will not ask for it. Abu-Saad (1984) found that Asian-American children tended to use words in the affective and evaluative domains (e.g., scary, sad, horrible, agonizing) when describing their pain. Nurses infer that Asian patients have less physical pain than other ethnic groups.

- African-American. Several studies have shown no difference between African-Americans and Caucasians in responses to pain.

- Hispanic. Hispanics tend to value stoicism. They think that difficulties should be borne with dignity and courage. They tend not to respond to early signs and symptoms. It is considered easier for women to seek treatment than men. Abu-Saad (1984) found that Latin-American children were more likely to use sensory words to describe pain (e.g., stinging, sore, burning, pumping). Nurses infer that Hispanic patients have the second greatest amount of pain of any ethnic group.

- Jewish. Jews tend to give dramatic accounts of pain experience, using adjectives such as "terrific" and "unbearable." They are also more pessimistic about the significance of pain. Nurses infer that Jews have the most physical and psychological pain of any ethnic group.

- Anglo-Saxon. Anglo-Saxons report pain with little emotion, and view pain as a defeated condition. Nurses infer that these patients will be stoic, second only to Asian patients.

Because culture affects the manner in which pain is communicated, nurses should not assess pain on the basis of the absence or presence of a particular behavior. Patients who might be called excessively emotional may just be manifesting behavioral characteristics of their culture. Having insight into cultural patterns of pain behavior can help nurses assess a patient's pain experience, but they must be aware that their own cultural biases can influence this assessment. Cultural aspects should be considered, but conclusions should not be based on these aspects alone.

Social Pressures

A person's pain behavior is not set in stone after childhood. Current circumstances can change it, sometimes quite dramatically. For example, one study (Craig, Best, & Reith, 1978) found that persons who observed another test subject exhibiting a low pain tolerance during an electric shock would subsequently have a lowered pain tolerance when receiving an identical shock. Conversely, if they observed a test subject highly tolerant of the electric shock, their subsequent pain tolerance increased significantly. This response is referred to as social modeling. It suggests that pain responses are not only subject to past learning but also exquisitely sensitive to the current environment.

Behavior Reinforcement

Like many other psychological and physiological responses, reinforcement of pain behaviors increases their intensity. That is, giving subjects greater attention if they express discomfort causes them to increase their pain behaviors and pain ratings. These observations have a great significance for the management of both acute and chronic pain. For example, reinforcement is a serious problem in chronic pain situations. The increased attention received by a family member when that member is in pain may serve as a reinforcer to the pain behaviors (e.g., wincing, complaining, limping).

Psychological Characteristics

Although many aspects of personality have been studied in relation to pain behaviors, only neuroticism and extroversion have consistently been associated with acute pain. Persons who are anxiety-prone or susceptible to excessive stress tend to react to stressful situations such as illness or trauma with more anxiety and thus may overreact to any pain associated with their ill health. These findings are not universal, however. At least two studies (Bond, 1984; Jacox, 1977) did not find a significant correlation between neuroticism, extroversion, and pain behavior.

A PSYCHOSOCIAL APPROACH TO PAIN MANAGEMENT

Patients come to clinics and hospitals with a lifetime of learning about how to behave when painfully ill or injured, what to expect from the health team, and what types of interventions will provide pain relief. Members of the health team need to gain some understanding of each patient's situation and belief system in order to provide optimal assistance.

How does the patient view his or her situation? What are the patient's beliefs about pain and its control? What is the patient's expectation of the health care team? For example, some patients may believe that only injectable analgesics can be effective against severe pain or that severe pain always means cancer. Others may think that all decisions about pain medications and doses should be made entirely by the health care team. Such beliefs, depending on their accuracy and how tenaciously the patient clings to them, can help or hinder attempts to provide health care.

SUMMARY

As clinicians have gained a better understanding of how strongly mental processes influence the pain experience, they have begun using more behavioral approaches to pain management. They no longer rely solely on chemical and surgical interventions. Perhaps the first behavioral pain control method to be used with a large number of patients was the Lamaze method of childbirth. In Lamaze classes, women learn a combination of behaviors they can use throughout labor and delivery to help reduce their perceptions of pain. Although using the behaviors does not make childbirth pain-free, it does decrease patients' anxiety and the total amount of analgesia and anesthesia used.

Research continues on how pain can be altered through behavioral interventions. The future promises many new and increasingly effective pain control methods that nurses will be using inside and outside the clinical setting.

EXAM QUESTIONS

Chapter 2

Questions 6–9

6. Which of the following is one of the cognitive influences on the pain experience?

   a. Intelligence
   b. Memory
   c. Anxiety
   d. Gender

7. What is defined as any medical treatment or nursing care that produces an effect in a patient because of its implicit or therapeutic intent, and not because of its specific nature?

   a. Placebo
   b. Controlled analgesia
   c. Reinforcement
   d. Social influence

8. In a group of 10 patients, how many will respond favorably to placebos at one time or another?

   a. 10
   b. 9
   c. 7
   d. 6

9. What is one of the social influences on the pain experience?

   a. Context
   b. Intelligence
   c. Anxiety
   d. Reinforcement

CHAPTER 3

THE PHYSIOLOGY OF PAIN

CHAPTER OBJECTIVE

After studying this chapter, the reader will be able to discuss the two major models of pain and the processes involved in pain conduction.

LEARNING OBJECTIVES

After studying this chapter, the reader will be able to

1. Specify the four steps in the conduction of pain impulses.

2. Describe the major differences between the intensity model and the gate control model of pain.

3. Describe the new intervention for pain relief that was introduced by the gate control theory of pain.

INTRODUCTION

The precise nature of pain has been the subject of speculation by philosophers, religious leaders, health care providers, and the lay public for many centuries. Among scientists and clinicians, two models of pain, sensory and intensity, remained prominent until 1965.

According to the sensory model, tissues have specific receptors for each type of sensation (e.g., temperature, touch, pressure), and each receptor responds only to a particular type of stimulation. For example, temperature receptors cannot respond to pressure, and pressure receptors cannot respond to temperature. In addition, in this model, the body has special transmission routes through the central nervous system and separate centers for reception and interpretation in the brain.

The intensity model arose from the observation that a stimulus of any kind, if great enough, can cause pain. For example, light pressure can be pleasurable, but intense pressure becomes painful. According to this model, pain is due to the intensity of the stimulus, not the type of stimulus. This model does not include receptors for specific types of pain. Rather, it holds that pain arises from stimuli that are strong enough to surpass an established pain threshold.

Today it is known that portions of each of these models are correct. Researchers have identified certain nerve fibers that are specific for pain. They have also discovered that stimulation of nonspecific nerve fibers gives rise to pain impulses, depending in part on the strength of the stimulus. One of the major drawbacks of the earlier models was that they ignored, or placed in a minor role, the impact of psychological factors. In 1965, Melzack and Wall proposed a new model, the gate control theory, that explains why and how psychological factors alter the amount of pain a person experiences.

THE GATE CONTROL THEORY

According to the gate control theory, the electrochemical impulses triggered by a noxious stimulus (e.g., a hammer hitting the thumb) to peripheral nerves can be modified or altered within the spinal cord itself, before the impulses reach the central nervous system. Melzack and Wall's revolutionary theory has held up well to years of research and remains the working model for pain researchers and clinicians throughout the world.

Simply stated, the gate control theory proposes that sensory nerves, composed of large and small fibers, constantly supply the brain with information from all areas of the body. Normal physical sensations travel along the larger fibers. The smaller fibers transmit pain impulses. All these fibers converge at a site in the dorsal horn of the spinal cord. This site is thought to act as a gating mechanism that determines which impulses are blocked and which are transmitted to the thalamus. The spinal gating mechanism is influenced by the relative number of impulses in large-diameter and small-diameter nerve fibers: Impulses in the large fibers tend to inhibit transmission (close the gate), whereas impulses in

the small fibers tend to facilitate it (open the gate). The gate is also influenced by nerve signals that descend from the brain. This gate mechanism is not an all-or-none phenomenon. The gate appears to be able to titrate the number of impulses allowed to pass through it.

The gate is responsive to a variety of influences, including a person's mood and level of anxiety. Positive moods close the gate, reducing the person's perception of pain. Negative emotions, such as fear and anxiety, open the gate, allowing pain impulses to be transmitted unchanged to the central nervous system. Other factors that affect the gating mechanism include a person's level of attentiveness, previous experiences, certain hormones, and concurrent presence of other strong stimuli.

Impact on Pain Management

Before the development of the gate control theory, pain interventions were based on models that maintained that the intensity of pain was determined by the intensity of the noxious stimulus applied and that the resulting pain sensations were transmitted directly and unchanged to the central nervous system. The only pain-reducing interventions suggested by these models were the following:

1. Eliminating the painful stimulus (e.g., by surgery, antibiotic therapy)

2. Blocking the pain pathways (e.g., by nerve blocks, analgesics)

3. Severing the nerve pathways

Unfortunately, these interventions often did not control pain. Particularly frustrating to health care teams were patients with chronic pain. One of the greatest benefits of the gate control theory was that it suggested new approaches to relieving both acute and chronic pain. Perhaps pain could be relieved by two approaches: reducing the transmission of pain impulses to the central nervous system by (1) using physical techniques and (2) altering the person's thought processes, emotions, or other behaviors. The new pain theory also promoted an interest in further research, particularly on the psychology of pain, an area that had been almost totally neglected.

CONDUCTION OF PAIN IMPULSES

Conduction of the pain signal consists of four steps: transduction, transmission, perception, and modulation. Transduction occurs when the chemical energy triggered by a noxious stimulus is changed to electrical activity in the endings of afferent nerve fibers (nociceptors). During transmission (Figure 3-1), the electrical impulses travel from peripheral nerve to spinal cord. Projection neurons then carry the message to the thalamus, and the message continues to the somatosensory cortex. The third step, perception, occurs in the cortex. Neural messages are converted into subjective experience. During the fourth step, modulation (Figure 3-2), a neural pathway in the central nervous system selectively inhibits transmission.

Each of the four steps has implications for treating pain. Understanding the physiology of pain conduc-

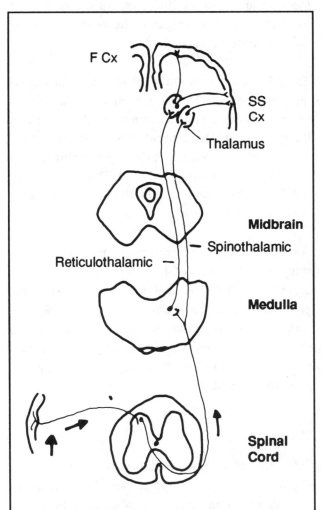

Figure 3-1. Transmission. *Source:* Reprinted with permission from Fields, 1987.

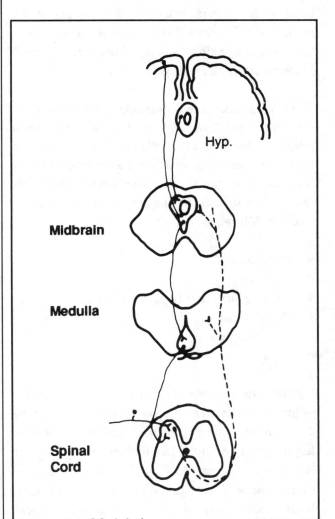

Figure 3-2. Modulation. *Source:* Reprinted with permission from Fields, 1987.

tion explains the rationale for the various pain-relieving interventions.

Transduction

Transduction, the step in which chemical energy is changed to electrical energy, generates an action potential in the neuron transmitting the pain signal. This is the peripheral pain system.

Primary afferent "pain" fibers or nociceptors are of two types: A delta fibers, which are myelinated and therefore transmit the signal fast, and C fibers, which are smaller and unmyelinated. This explains the two types of pain felt with an injury. For example, when a bump to the ankle occurs, an initial sharp pain is felt immediately (A delta fibers). This is followed by a throbbing achy pain (C fibers). C fibers are involved in longer lasting, chronic pain.

The afferent fibers are activated by any noxious stimulus (mechanical, thermal, or chemical) that causes release of biochemical mediators. These mediators lead to generation of an action potential and electrical changes in the neuron. Biochemical mediators that activate or sensitize the nociceptive response include the following:

- Potassium
- Histamine
- Neurotransmitters (e.g., substance P)
- Prostaglandins
- Leukotrienes
- Bradykinin

Possible interventions at this step include inhibition of prostaglandins. These compounds are released by damaged cells. Some of the nonopioid analgesics (referred to as nonsteroidal antiinflammatory drugs, or NSAIDs) are potent blockers of prostaglandins. Another possible intervention is use of membrane stabilizers, anticonvulsants, or anesthetics that prevent the generation of an action potential in the neuron. Examples of these are carbamazepine, mexiletine,

and lidocaine. By preventing transduction, the pain signal is stopped at the peripheral level, so the experience of pain is not realized.

Transmission

During transmission, the nociceptive signal travels along the afferent fibers, terminating in the dorsal horn of the spinal cord. Neuropeptides and other substances are released from the neuron, primarily substance P. Substance P is thought to diffuse to secondary neurons, where it binds with receptor sites, triggering an action potential. These secondary neurons, called spinothalamic tract neurons, carry the signal to the contralateral side of the spinal cord. Most terminate in the thalamus; some terminate in the midbrain. This synapse is the proposed gate in the gate control theory of pain.

The primary intervention at the transmission stage is the use of opioids. These drugs bind to opiate receptor sites on the afferent neuron in the dorsal horn of the spinal cord. This prevents release of neurotransmitters such as substance P, thereby stopping the signal at the level of the spinal cord. This explains why opioids work so well intraspinally or epidurally. They are delivered to the site of action.

Another possible intervention at this step is cordotomy. Because the fibers involved in transmission occur in a well-defined region in the spinal cord, the pain message can be inhibited by ablating the tract surgically. This procedure is saved for patients with a short life expectancy, because the fibers may regenerate, or fibers that normally do not transmit pain may become activated.

Perception

Perception of pain occurs in the cortex. Fibers from the thalamus transmit the nociceptive message to several areas in the cortex: the somatosensory cortex (associated with the intensity and quality of pain) and the association cortex (associated with affective types of pain), both in the parietal lobe, and the limbic system (associated with anxiety). It is at this stage that persons realize that they are hurting. It is the least understood of all the stages in pain conduction.

Modulation

The body has its own ability to change the pain signal. The fibers that terminate in the midbrain stimulate regions that send descending signals to the dorsal horn of the spinal cord. These neurons inhibit the transmission of nociception by releasing substances such as serotonin and norepinephrine. Endogenous opiates (endorphins) also play a role in modulation. They bind to the afferent neuron and prevent the release of substance P in the same way as exogenously administered narcotics.

Interventions at this step include activities that may increase the level of endorphins (e.g., transcutaneous electrical nerve stimulation [TENS], hypnosis). Because norepinephrine is present as a neurotransmitter in the descending fibers, clonidine, a noradrenergic antagonist, has been used epidurally and intraspinally. Pain is relieved with this drug, but the hypotensive effects are significant. Other noradrenergic antagonists with less effect on the cardiovascular system are under investigation. Another possible intervention is use of tricyclic antidepressants. Antidepressants inhibit the reuptake of serotonin into the descending neuron, which allows more serotonin to be available in the synaptic cleft.

SUMMARY

Theories about the physiological basis of pain have included the sensory and intensity models. The current model, the gate control theory, provides a physiological basis that can be used to explain why and how psychological factors alter the perception of pain. Conduction of the pain signal has four steps: transduction, transmission, perception, and modulation. An understanding of each of these steps makes it possible to plan different approaches to interventions for pain relief.

EXAM QUESTIONS

Chapter 3

Questions 10–15

10. What model of pain suggests that pain can be caused by stimulation of any receptors if the stimulation is strong enough to surpass the established pain threshold?

    a. Sensory model
    b. Intensity model
    c. Gate control model
    d. Threshold model

11. What model of pain proposes that electrochemical impulses from the peripheral nerves can be modified or altered within the spinal cord itself, before the impulses reach the central nervous system?

    a. Sensory model
    b. Intensity model
    c. Gate control model
    d. Threshold model

12. Which of the four steps in the conduction of the pain signal constitutes an energy change from chemical to electrical?

    a. Modulation
    b. Perception
    c. Transmission
    d. Transduction

13. Which of the following pain-reducing interventions was introduced by the gate control theory of pain?

    a. Eliminating the painful stimulus
    b. Severing nerve pathways
    c. Altering the patient's emotions
    d. Blocking the pain pathways

14. At which of the four steps in pain conduction can opioids bind to receptor sites to stop the pain signal at the level of the spinal cord?

    a. Modulation
    b. Perception
    c. Transmission
    d. Transduction

15. At what anatomical site does perception of pain occur?

    a. Dorsal horn of the spinal cord
    b. Nociceptors
    c. Thalamus
    d. Cortex

CHAPTER 4

ASSESSMENT OF PAIN

CHAPTER OBJECTIVE

After studying this chapter, the reader will be able to recognize components, tools, and guidelines for physical assessment of patients with pain and the attitudes that patients and health care professionals may have toward pain.

LEARNING OBJECTIVES

After studying this chapter, the reader will be able to

1. Explain why many health professionals think they know more about pain than their patients do.

2. Recognize one of the two major reasons health care professionals are afraid to trust patients to evaluate the severity of the patients' own pain.

3. Specify two reasons patients who have pain may not show any distress.

4. Explain why a patient who has pain may still be able to sleep.

5. Recognize the components of a thorough physical assessment of a patient who has

pain and the reasons for repeated assessments.

6. Indicate a useful tool that can be used to assess the severity of pain.

INTRODUCTION

Inadequate control of pain invariably begins with improper assessment of the patient. This chapter describes common myths that interfere with accurate assessment of pain, examines the nurse's influential role in pain management, and discusses the proper methods of assessing pain. This is the first step in the nursing process in caring for a patient in pain. The nursing diagnoses for pain are also discussed.

MYTHS THAT INTERFERE WITH PAIN ASSESSMENT

Both nurses and patients have misconceptions about pain that interfere with the ability to adequately assess and manage it. These misconceptions are the result of pain-related experiences throughout life inside and outside the workplace. Nurses may not be aware of their misconceptions, but every nurse has some.

Pain assessment depends on accurate communication between patients and health care professionals. Inadequate assessment is virtually assured if either or both of the following problems occur:

1. Staff personnel misread the pain signals being sent by the patient.

2. The patient sends out mixed messages because he or she misunderstands what staff personnel need to see or be told in order to be convinced that the pain is "real."

Problems in communication usually result from myths that both groups have about pain. The most common and troublesome of these myths are discussed in the following section.

MYTH: Health Care Professionals Are the Authorities on a Patient's Pain

The myth that health care professionals are the authorities on a patient's pain underlies nearly all problems in the effective treatment of pain. In her myth-busting book on pain management, McCaffery (1979) asks: Who is the authority about the patient's pain—the health team or the patient? Too many health care professionals think that they know more about a patient's pain than the patient does. They seem to think that they, not the person in pain, can best decide if pain exists, and if they decide that the patient is having pain, they then go on to decide how severe the pain is.

Another nurse specializing in pain management also noted serious deficiencies in the way nurses respond to patients having pain:

> [The responses] can still be described as limited, automatic, and reflective of the nurse's private experiences and opinions. There are

exceptions, of course, but in this author's experience in a variety of locations, the need to improve nurse response to pain is still an urgent one. Failure to recognize the unique nature of the pain experience is expressed in the typical comment, "I've had pain myself and I know you don't have to carry on as that patient is doing." "I don't care what you say, I know she just wants attention" reflects another common belief. Pain is judged to be "real" or not, or to be a bid for a narcotic "high," and the nurses continue to reduce analgesic dosage for fear of causing addiction. (Graffam, 1982)

Where do health professionals get the idea that they know more about a patient's pain than the patient does? McCaffery suggests that part of the reason for this idea is the inability to measure pain. Pain cannot be measured objectively, and there is no way to determine if it actually exists. This makes health professionals uncomfortable, because it means they must trust the patient to tell them when pain is present and if their interventions have been effective. Furthermore, professional authority, which is supported in part by the ability to measure and interpret physiological abnormalities (e.g., pulse rates, blood and urine tests, electrocardiograms), is threatened when a disorder cannot be measured.

Trusting a patient to evaluate the severity of his or her own pain is frightening to health professionals for two reasons. First, they fear that the patient may be a malingerer. That is, they worry that the patient is trying to deceive them, is only pretending to feel pain in order to avoid or gain something. This fear is certainly not irrational, particularly for professionals working with patients who may have monetary reasons for faking pain. Most health professionals are aware of instances in which injuries were exaggerated in personal injury cases to increase the amount of the settlement. However, true malingerers account for only a small proportion of patients being seen for the treatment of pain.

Second, they fear that the patient may be exaggerating an existing pain (consciously or unconsciously) in order to dull psychological distress or simply get attention in the form of medical or surgical treatment. No health professional wants to aid or abet these destructive coping mechanisms.

Generally, only two approaches are feasible when a patient complains of pain. One is to assume that most patients complaining of pain are experiencing pain caused by physiological problems. Operating under this assumption, the health professional treats the pain with appropriate doses or types of analgesics and other measures. When this approach is used, malingerers or patients with psychosomatic disorders sometimes receive inappropriate treatments.

The second approach is based on two mistaken assumptions: (1) a lot of patients are malingerers or hysterics and are trying to get treatment for nonexistent or exaggerated pain, and (2) it is worse to treat malingerers and hysterics with potent analgesics than it is to withhold treatment from patients who really have pain. When this approach is used, many patients with pain will suffer unnecessarily.

In reality, most health professionals alternate between these two approaches. If they think a patient is believable, the patient's pain is treated. If the patient is judged to be suspect, then treatment is often confined to safe pain-relief measures (e.g., heat, aspirin, rest), even for patients complaining of moderate or severe pain.

Certainly, not every patient who complains of pain should be treated with potent opioids. This would be too simplistic. However, constantly being concerned that a potent opioid may be prescribed for a patient who is malingering or has a psychosomatic disorder is also not a reasonable approach. The key to preventing long-term problems in pain management is proper assessment of the pain, followed by adequate treatment and adequate follow-up. More problems

with chronic pain are started by undertreatment of acute pain than by overtreatment.

MYTH: The Patient's Pain Can Always Be Verified by Characteristic Behaviors and Physiological Changes

Health care professionals expect patients with moderate or severe pain to behave in certain ways and have specific physiological changes (Table 4-1). These changes are due to the activation of the sympathetic and parasympathetic nervous systems, the flight-or-fight response.

Despite the presence of severe pain, patients often do not show these expected signs or behaviors. The human body cannot maintain a high state of readiness indefinitely. After a time, usually a few weeks, the body physiologically adapts to the pain, and the characteristic physiological and behavioral responses disappear. In their place often appear behavioral changes such as depression and lethargy (behaviors not usually thought of as associated with moderate or severe pain).

Health care professionals who are not aware of the underlying connection between prolonged pain and depression may decide that the patient's pain is gone (or was never really present) and that the underlying problem has always been depression. At this point, the patient may be deprived of any potent analgesics and placed on antidepressants.

Pain Etiquette

Everyone has expectations about how and when pain should be expressed. However, as discussed in chapter 2, ways of expressing pain differ from person to person. In some cultures, pain displays such as moaning, grimacing, or verbally complaining are considered shameful. To maintain their favorable self-concept, patients from these cultures may make every effort to suppress overt expressions of pain. This is particularly true when health professionals reinforce this stoic behavior (You're such a good pa-

---

TABLE 4-1
Acute Pain Response Model

Physiological Responses

- Increased pulse rate, blood pressure, respiratory rate and depth
- Dilated pupils, increased perspiration, nausea, pallor
- Decreased urinary output
- Decreased peristalsis of gastrointestinal tract
- Increased basal metabolic rate

Behavioral Responses

- Body activity decreased
- Protection of painful areas
- Facial expression exhibits fear, distress, or other negative emotions
- Verbal expressions such as moaning, groaning

---

tient, hardly ever complaining. You should hear some of our other patients.).

Patients with chronic pain have some of the greatest difficulty in communicating their distress to others. Many of these patients do not want to complain constantly about their pain. Yet, staff personnel expect some ongoing signs of distress before they feel comfortable in administering additional medication. Members of the nursing staff are adept at using facial expressions, comments, and withdrawal to let patients know that pain complaints are not believed. Patients having a great deal of pain are then forced into behaviors they may find demeaning in order to get sufficient pain relief. McCaffery (1979) warns nurses:

> If we find ourselves doubting the patient's statement that he has pain because his other behavior does not verify its presence, it is instructive to ask ourselves, How would this patient have to behave in order for me to believe him? Sometimes we then discover that the behavior we expect to see might be embarrassing to the patient or actually maladaptive.

Several years ago a physician consulted a nurse on the hospital's pain management team about a cancer patient. Despite numerous increases in pain medications, the patient continued to complain of severe pain. However, members of the nursing staff told the physician that the patient's pain was better.

To clarify the current situation, the nurse from the pain management team talked with the patient and the nursing staff. Then she carefully studied the nursing notes and medication records. Eventually, she determined that the nursing staff had not been giving the patient the increasing doses of narcotics the physician had been ordering (the nurses had been allowed to select a dose from a range and to administer the narcotics as needed). The nursing staff was not uncaring. What had caused them to undermedicate this patient? The patient was terminal and certainly appeared to be alert.

A discussion with the nursing staff revealed that they did not think the patient was in as much pain as he told his doctor. They all thought his pain was not very severe because he walked rapidly up and down the hallway for hours each shift. After receiving his dose of medication, he would go to bed and sleep for awhile and then start his race again. To the nursing staff, the patient's behavior was inconsistent with his complaints.

In talks with the pain specialist, the patient revealed that when his pain became severe he walked rapidly in an attempt to distract himself. The unfortunate outcome was that the more active he became, the less pain medication his nurses gave him. Only if he had stayed in bed and acted the way patients in pain were **supposed to** would the nurses have believed his complaints. Once the nurses became aware of why he was pacing the hallways and he was put on a regular dose of opioid analgesic, his pain was controlled.

MYTH: The Presence of Sleep Means the Absence of Pain

Another time when normal behavioral responses to moderate or severe pain are obliterated is when the patient is sleeping because of overwhelming fatigue. This happens often on the intensive care unit (ICU). Constant monitoring and treatments and the incessant noise and light make normal sleep nearly impossible. Unfortunately, staff personnel tend to assume that any patient who is asleep must no longer be in severe pain. Patients' dozing off between interruptions is commonly interpreted by nurses and physicians as the absence of pain rather than the presence of exhaustion.

Similar situations occur regularly outside the ICU, of course. Patients who have been caught sleeping are not believed when they complain of severe pain upon awakening. Nurses need to be aware that patients can sleep despite considerable pain if sufficiently tired. A patient should never be refused a pain medication because he or she was asleep a few minutes before.

MYTH: If the Cause of Pain Cannot Be Identified, It Is Not Real Pain

Not too many years ago, menstrual cramps were considered imaginary and the result of psychological problems. Now, it is known that the painful cramps felt by hundreds of thousands of women each year are very real and are due to uterine anoxia (i.e., angina of the uterus). Although the disorder may be exacerbated by a variety of factors, the pain itself is caused by prolonged uterine contractions.

The list of painful diseases previously thought to be imaginary is long, and thousands of case histories provide examples of instances in which the causes of "imaginary" pains were only discovered at autopsy. As medicine continues to become more sophisticated, physiological explanations likely will be found for many of the painful conditions that are still thought to be all in the patient's head. Nevertheless, many health professionals continue to assume that if no physical disorder can be found to explain a patient's pain, then the pain must be imaginary. This places the patient in a distressing situation: not only does the pain have no explanation or adequate treatment, but the patient is supposed to stop feeling the pain because it is not really there. For the patient's emotional and physical well-being, it is nearly always preferable for the health team to assume that the patient is having pain for which an explanation has not yet been found, rather than to assume that the pain is not real.

Concern about the possible development of chronic pain problems is appropriate only after pain has been present for more than a month. At this point, a different approach to pain treatment should be considered. Before this point, the treatment for pain of unknown origin should be the same as that for a disorder that can be totally eliminated (e.g., appendicitis) or minimized through treatment (e.g., tennis elbow). When pain becomes chronic, particularly in cases in which the patient is not terminally ill, the situation becomes much more complex. A consultation with a pain specialist is recommended to avoid a situation in which the pain and disability continue to escalate. If the patient is terminally ill, another set of problems must be addressed to avoid problems in pain management.

MYTH: Patients' Denial of Pain Problems Means There Is No Pain or the Pain Is Being Controled

Patients do not always reveal the presence or the true severity of their pain. The reasons for downplaying symptoms are complex. June L. Dahl, a pain expert and professor of pharmacology at the University of Wisconsin, recently remarked, "Many patients fear that if they focus too much attention on the subject [of pain] they will alienate [their caregivers] or take [their doctors'] precious time away from their diseases" (Roark, 1991).

Another reason for not admitting to a pain problem is related to what patients think the pain means about their well-being. They may fear that the pain means they have cancer or some other life-threatening disease. Others who already know that they have a potentially fatal disease may equate pain severity with disease severity. They try to avoid hearing bad news by denying or understating a pain problem. Denial of significant pain can also be used by patients to avoid other realities, such as worrying family members, being prohibited from doing certain activities (e.g., playing a sport), or being thought a sissy. Health professionals need to watch for other indications of pain (e.g., decreased appetite, avoidance of certain movements, limping).

EFFECTIVE ASSESSMENT OF PAIN

Proper treatment of pain requires a proper assessment. Ideally, the outcome of a thorough assessment is detection of the source of pain and corrective therapy, thus eliminating the problem. Unfortunately, complete pain relief is not always possible, particularly in the short term.

The basic approach to pain assessment is listed in Table 4-2. Although the initial assessment is usually performed by a physician, nurses may sometimes be responsible for collecting the information and communicating it to a physician. The thoroughness of this initial work-up depends in large part on the patient's condition. For instance, a patient who is in obvious distress and complaining of severe chest pain will not be asked in-depth questions for a medical history before diagnostic procedures are started to rule out any life-threatening conditions. When time allows, the diagnostic process begins with the approach described in the following sections.

Initial assessments are done to determine underlying disease. Repeated assessments are performed for other important reasons:

- To determine if the underlying disease (the cause of the patient's pain) is responding to treatment or progressing

- To detect the presence of complications related to the disease or to treatment

- To determine the adequacy of pain control interventions

Because they spend the most time with patients and administer most of the pain treatments, nurses are often responsible for assessing the severity of pain to determine if the pain is being adequately controlled.

TABLE 4-2
Physical Assessment of Pain

Initial Onset of the Pain and Any Accompanying Symptoms

- Location, radiation of pain (starts one place and spreads to another)
- Severity of pain
- Characteristics of pain (sharp, dull, etc.)
- Relationship to other events: meals, bowel or bladder function, physical activity

Course of the Pain Progress and Evolution of All the Symptoms

- Past and present status of pain and accompanying symptoms
- Which activities, movements make the pain better or worse
- Effect of pain on activities of daily living

The following section explains step-by-step how to do this assessment effectively.

Location of the Pain

It is not necessary to determine the location of the patient's pain each time additional analgesia is given. However, it is necessary to check at regular intervals that both the nurse and the patient are talking about the same pain (e.g., Are you still having that pain in your abdomen?).

One reason for regularly determining the location of the pain is that sometimes a new source of discomfort develops, and the patient does not know that the change should be mentioned. These intermittent assessments are particularly important when patients are self-medicating by using patient-controlled analgesia (PCA). When a new pain develops, these patients tend to respond by giving themselves more medication. The new pain, however, may be better treated by another method (e.g., catheterization for bladder distension or anesthetic throat sprays for postoperative sore throats caused by intubation).

Even more worrisome, changes in the pattern, intensity, or location of the patient's pain may be the ear-

liest indication that a complication is developing. For instance, a patient with abdominal pain reports having pain in a new area, the supraclavicular regions, that is made worse by taking a deep breath. This new pain could be a signal that intraperitoneal bleeding or infection is irritating the diaphragm (with pain referred to the shoulder region). The patient, sedated and unaware of the new pain's significance, may not mention this new symptom unless asked about the location of his or her pain. This information can be obtained by asking the patient to point to the areas where he or she is experiencing pain.

Pain arising from structures deep in the body (e.g., the gallbladder or heart) occurs both at the site of the organ concerned and at other distant sites. A familiar example is the referral of cardiac pain into the left arm or the left side of the jaw. Another example is pain in the anterior aspect of the right shoulder that occurs in patients with inflammation of the gallbladder.

Referred pain is experienced in the regions of the body supplied by the same nerve roots as the diseased organ (Bonica, 1987). That is, the sites and the organ are supplied by the same dermatome (Figure

Referred pain is experienced in the regions of the body supplied by the same nerve roots as the diseased organ (Bonica, 1987). That is, the sites and the organ are supplied by the same dermatome (Figure 4-1). The underlying mechanism appears to be the opening of the spinal gate (lowering the threshold to the transmission of painful sensations) at the level of the spinal cord where the impulses are received from the involved dermatome. The threshold is lowered so completely that even the skin in the area of referred pain becomes hypersensitive (hyperesthetic), and the slightest touch feels painful to the patient.

Patterns of pain referral are so consistent that they have considerable diagnostic value. For example, a child with a "stomachache" points to the umbilical region when asked where it hurts. The physician immediately suspects appendicitis, even though the appendix is located more in the right lower quadrant.

The Intensity and Other Characteristics of Pain

The intensity of pain is often the most difficult characteristic to assess accurately. Patients find it difficult to judge the severity of their own pain and may deny its severity for other reasons.

Although several sophisticated tools are available for assessing the intensity and quality of pain, they are used most appropriately in cases of chronic pain. An easy-to-use tool for measuring the intensity of acute pain is available (Figure 4-2). This simple tool uses a scale of 0 to 10, with 0 indicating no pain and 10 indicating the worst pain the patient can imagine.

This tool can be used in almost any setting, as long as the patient understands English and is sufficiently alert to comprehend the questions. A printed pain chart or visual analogue scale is not necessary to use the tool. The advantage of this numeric method is that it provides patients a way to communicate the severity of their pain without using imprecise words such as "terrible," "bad," or "better." The tool also provides the nurse with a number indicating pain intensity that can be used for comparison in future assessments of the patient's pain.

A few patients cannot understand the concept of using numbers to describe the intensity of their pain. In such instances, words will have to suffice (Figure 4-2). It can also be helpful to have the patient use at least two descriptive words: one that indicates how severe the pain is and another that indicates whether it is getting better or worse.

The key in using pain intensity scales is to consistently use the same scale. A rating of 5 will mean something entirely different on a 0 to 10 scale than it does on a 0 to 5 scale. The scale being used should be indicated in the nursing care plan, in order to ensure consistency.

Pain comes in many different types, and patients are often at a loss to describe to others what they are feeling (see "The Language of Pain" in chapter 1). The McGill-Melzack Pain Questionnaire (Appendix A) contains a list of words that can be used to help patients better describe their pain. Also, some persons use the word "pain" only to describe severe discomfort. If a patient denies that he or she is having pain, rephrasing questions so that the word "discomfort" replaces the word "pain" may be helpful.

In addition to the intensity of pain, the clinician also needs to determine what makes the pain better or worse. This can sometimes be accomplished by direct questions: "Have you noticed anything you do that seems to make the pain better or worse?" Information obtained in this manner can be extremely useful.

Sometimes the information must be obtained by observing the patient's behavior. Patients may be totally unaware that they are doing things to reduce their pain. For example, patients with pain caused by pancreatitis or inflammation of the gallbladder may sit in a characteristic position: leaning forward so that the inflamed organ does not rest against the posterior wall of the abdomen. They are usually unaware that they are using the position to decrease the pain.

Common Locations of Referred Pain
AREAS OF VISCERAL REFERRED PAIN
(Posterior Aspect)

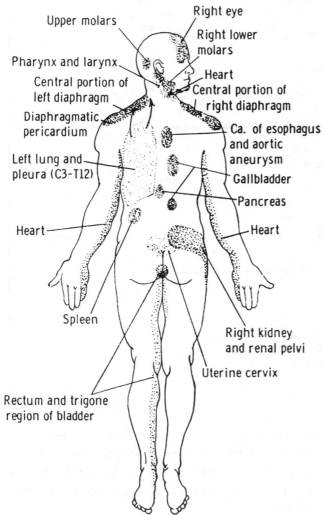

Upper molars

Right eye

Right lower molars

Pharynx and larynx

Central portion of left diaphragm

Heart

Central portion of right diaphragm

Diaphragmatic pericardium

Ca. of esophagus and aortic aneurysm

Left lung and pleura (C3-T12)

Gallbladder

Pancreas

Heart

Heart

Spleen

Right kidney and renal pelvi

Uterine cervix

Rectum and trigone region of bladder

Common Locations of Referred Pain
AREAS OF VISCERAL REFERRED PAIN
(Anterior Aspect)

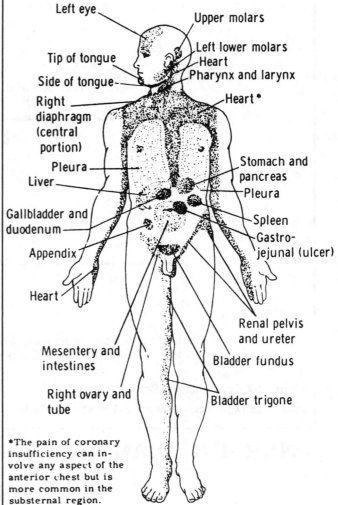

Left eye

Upper molars

Left lower molars

Heart

Tip of tongue

Side of tongue

Pharynx and larynx

Right diaphragm (central portion)

Heart *

Pleura

Liver

Stomach and pancreas

Pleura

Gallbladder and duodenum

Spleen

Gastro-jejunal (ulcer)

Appendix

Heart

Renal pelvis and ureter

Bladder fundus

Mesentery and intestines

Right ovary and tube

Bladder trigone

*The pain of coronary insufficiency can involve any aspect of the anterior chest but is more common in the substernal region.

A

B

Figure 4-1 . Common locations of referred pain.

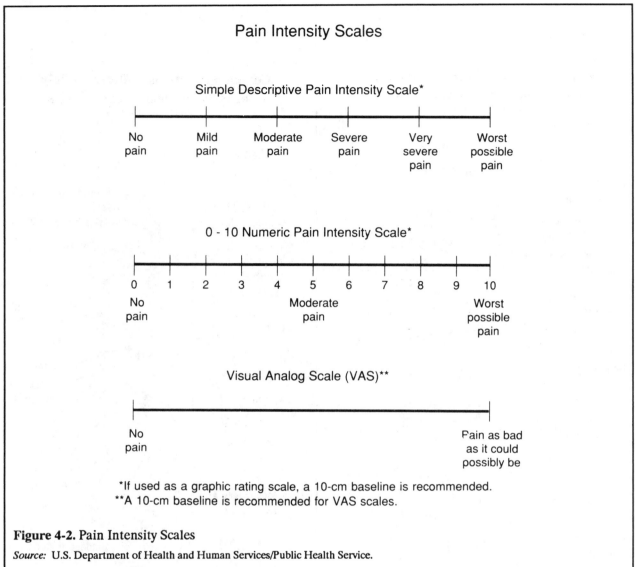

Figure 4-2. Pain Intensity Scales

Source: U.S. Department of Health and Human Services/Public Health Service.

NURSING DIAGNOSES

Two diagnoses are used in diagnosing pain: pain and chronic pain. These diagnoses are defined by the time frames indicated in chapter 1.

The etiology for the diagnostic statement must be one that nursing interventions can change. Therefore, "pain related to surgery" would be inappropriate. No nursing intervention could change the fact that the patient had surgery. Instead, the nursing in-

terventions are aimed toward the effects that the surgery had on the patient. "Pain related to the effects of surgery" captures the nursing process more succinctly.

Related nursing diagnoses include anxiety, disturbance in sleep pattern, activity intolerance, powerlessness, fear, impaired physical mobility, and ineffective individual coping. This list is not all-inclusive. Which diagnoses apply will depend on the effects the pain is having on the patient.

SUMMARY

Several myths or misconceptions about pain can interfere with the accurate assessment of pain and effective pain treatment. Important pain characteristics that need to be assessed and documented include the location of the pain, the intensity and type of pain, and alleviating and aggravating factors. Regular assessments are needed, and tools are available that can help in obtaining accurate assessments. The nursing diagnoses for patients in pain are pain and chronic pain. Important guidelines for the effective treatment of pain are presented in chapter 5 along with the relative advantages and disadvantages of various methods for treating pain.

EXAM QUESTIONS

Chapter 4

Questions 16–23

16. According to McCaffery, why do many health professionals think that they know more about patients' pain than the patients do?

    a. Little experience with pain themselves
    b. Inability to measure pain
    c. Insecurity about giving opioids
    d. The high number of addicted patients

17. Many patients who have a great deal of pain do not act as if they are distressed. Why is this?
    a. More opioids are given to patients who do not complain.
    b. They have been told the pain cannot be relieved.
    c. Their pain thresholds are higher than those of most persons.
    d. They do not want to complain constantly.

18. Why do many patients who are having a great deal of pain deny it or downplay the severity of it?

    a. They have an extreme fear of opioid addiction.
    b. They avoid any kind of injections.
    c. Their families become angry when the patients admit to pain.
    d. They think more severe pain means more severe disease.

19. If pain suddenly develops in a patient who has not had pain previously, what information should be gather before the physician is called?

    a. Location of the pain and preferred route of administration of medications
    b. Location, severity, and characteristics of the pain
    c. Patient's speculations about why he or she is having pain
    d. Any information about previous serious drug problems

20. Which of the following is a useful tool for assessing the severity of pain that almost all clinicians can use?

    a. Numeric pain intensity scale
    b. Acute pain monitor
    c. The Gate Scale
    d. Pressure detection monitor

21. Which of the following statements explains why many health care professionals do not trust patients to evaluate the severity of the patients' own pain?

    a. They think patients are incapable of assessing pain.
    b. They know that many people become irrational with pain.
    c. They think that patients do not know when medication is needed.
    d. They fear that patients may exaggerate existing pain.

22. If a patient who has been sleeping soundly wakes up and complains of pain, what should the nurse assume?

    a. The patient is a malingerer.
    b. The opioid is too good to resist.
    c. Anxiety, not pain, is the problem.
    d. The patient was sleeping because he or she was exhausted.

23. What is one purpose of repeated assessments of pain for a hospitalized patient?

    a. To ensure that the patient is not malingering
    b. To protect the nursing staff from litigation
    c. To detect the presence of drug addiction
    d. To monitor the progression of disease

CHAPTER 5

APPROACHES TO PAIN MANAGEMENT

CHAPTER OBJECTIVE

After studying this chapter, the reader will be able to discuss guidelines and techniques used to relieve pain and their various advantages and disadvantages.

LEARNING OBJECTIVES

After studying this chapter, the reader will be able to

1. Name two of the three guidelines for improving pain relief.

2. Specify one invasive technique that can be used for pain control and one major disadvantage for its use.

3. Specify major advantages for using applications of heat and cold to reduce muscle spasm and pain.

4. Select a noninvasive technique that can be used for pain control.

INTRODUCTION

Little that physicians and nurses do is more important than relieving pain. Yet, study after study shows that the treatment of pain, both inside and outside the hospital, continues to be inadequate. This failure is due in part to the medical system's strong orientation toward treating the disease rather than the patient (and the patient's signs and symptoms). As a result of this orientation, physicians and nurses receive relatively little formal training or reinforcement in the clinical setting for controlling patients' signs and symptoms.

A recent survey (Graffam, 1990) of 4-year nursing programs showed that on average, nursing students receive only 1.4 hr of instruction on beliefs and misconceptions about pain and 3.9 hr on the use of analgesics. In light of the amount of time nurses spend controlling pain, the briefness of their education on pain management is difficult to reconcile. Anna Omrey, a specialist in nursing ethics at the University of California, Los Angeles, noted that the issue of pain control has become the number one "ethical dilemma" concerning nurses (Roark, 1991).

Nursing is not the only profession lacking adequate education on pain. Bonica (1990) reviewed 10 textbooks on medicine and surgery and 11 on oncology published in the United States. These are the standard texts for medical students, house officers, and practitioners throughout the country. In a total of almost 27,000 pages, only 162 (0.6%) addressed symptomatic treatment of acute and chronic pain.

This chapter provides basic information on the interventions commonly used to relieve pain inside and outside the clinical setting. Because of the complexity of the pain experience, a variety of measures should be used to relieve a patient's pain.

ANALGESICS

One of the most commonly used methods of treating pain is administration of analgesics, drugs that reduce the perception of pain. This section discusses the various ways analgesics can be used to manage pain. The underlying mechanisms by which these chemicals interfere with pain are considered in chapter 6.

Routes of Administration

Analgesics can be administered by a variety of routes. The most common routes are oral, intramuscular, and intravenous. Less common ones are subcutaneous, rectal, sublingual, transdermal, intrapleural, and intrathecal.

The manner in which analgesics are administered is also variable. For example, cancer patients with consistent, severe pain require large doses of opioids. A growing number of these patients can be ambulatory nowadays thanks to the development of miniaturized infusion pumps that administer drugs on a continuous basis. The medication is infused through a permanent indwelling catheter. The catheter is inserted into a large vein or into the intrathecal or epidural spaces within the spinal canal.

Another infusion device, called the Ommaya reservoir, can be implanted under the skin. With this device, analgesics (or chemotherapeutic agents) can be delivered directly into the patient's intrathecal or epidural spaces or even directly into a ventricle of the brain. The use of intraventricular analgesics is still experimental, however.

Implantable continuous infusion devices and the surgical procedure used to implant them are expensive. As a result, only those patients whose pain is not responsive to conventional analgesic therapy and who are expected to live for more than a few months are generally considered candidates for implanted pumps (McQuire, 1987).

Pumps that allow patients to initiate additional doses of intravenous analgesics are also growing in popularity. Called patient-controlled analgesia (PCA), this method is effective in controlling moderate to severe pain. PCA is discussed in greater detail later in the textbook.

Guidelines for Use

The following questions and answers cover some common concerns about the use of analgesics for acute pain.

Q: Should patients be encouraged to wait until their pain is more than mild or moderate before they request more pain medication? And how much should they be given? Enough to "take the edge off" their pain or enough to relieve their pain completely?

A: Two myths about the treatment of acute pain seem to be nearly universal: (1) use of potent analgesics should be delayed as long as possible and (2) the doses of these drugs should be as small as possible.

Many persons, including health professionals, think that the use of strong analgesics should be delayed as long as possible because patients who receive a lot of opiod analgesics can become addicted. However, surveys of thousands of patients treated with opioid analgesics for moderate to severe pain have found no cases of addiction. (Addiction is discussed more thoroughly in chapter 7.)

A good reason for not delaying an additional dose of pain medication is that it is easier to relieve the pain while the pain is still mild. Waiting until the pain is worse will increase the amount of analgesic required and the amount of time it takes for the patient to become comfortable again.

One reason given for administering only enough analgesic to "take the edge off" a patient's pain is that when potent pain medications are used "too soon" (i.e., too early in the course of a disease), the patient will become tolerant to opioids and then "nothing will be strong enough" to treat the pain when it gets

worse in the future. This fear is based on the mistaken belief that there is a maximum dose of opioid that can be given to a patient. In fact, the amount of opioid that can be administered has no "ceiling." No patient should be left uncomfortable because of fear of being unable to control future discomfort.

The objective of administering analgesics is to make patients comfortable. If pain is allowed to continue, a vicious cycle can be started. Unrelieved pain leads to increases in the patient's anxiety and increases in muscle tension. The anxiety and muscle tension then lead to more pain (Figure 5-1). Therefore, the goal in treating pain should always be to make the patient relaxed. This does not mean heavy sedation. The

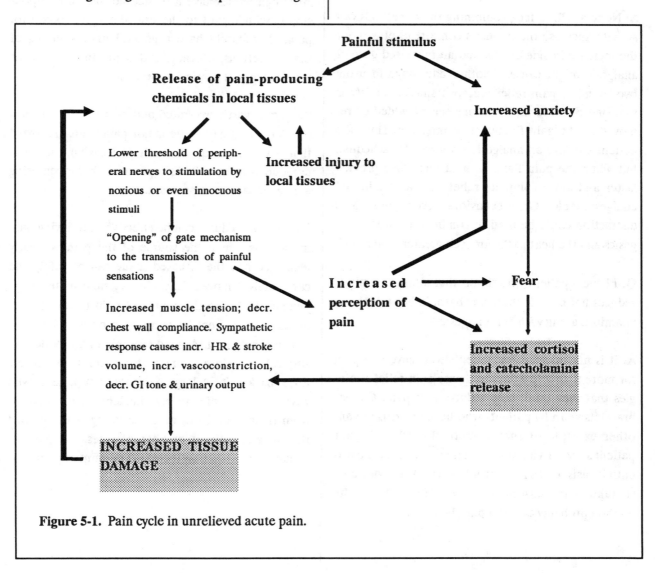

Figure 5-1. Pain cycle in unrelieved acute pain.

dose given should provide pain relief without excessive side effects.

Nurses can help prevent the establishment of a pain cycle by educating patients about the hazards of waiting too long to request or take analgesics or use other pain-relieving measures. Hospitalized patients should be instructed to inform their nurses when pain is beginning to return. Patients on PCA should be taught to inject additional analgesic when they first notice the pain returning, not to wait until they "can't take it any more."

Q: Are there any problems with combining analgesics with other types of pain relief?

A: None at all. In fact, combining these methods can actually increase the patient's comfort level without the increase in side effects that an increased dose of analgesic might cause. Another advantage in using two or more pain-relief methods simultaneously is that one or more interventions can be added or removed as the pain fluctuates in intensity. Thus, the patient can use an analgesic on a regular schedule, but when the pain flares, a heat pack may provide faster and more complete relief than an additional analgesic tablet. Or, a behavioral technique such as distraction could be used in combination with analgesics and the heat packs for even greater pain relief.

Q: I have a patient who thinks that taking vitamin C reduces her pain. Is there any harm in her taking the vitamin C along with her analgesics?

A: It is not unusual for patients who have had pain for more than a few days to devise pain-relief strategies that they think help reduce their pain. Copper bracelets worn by patients who have arthritis are another example of such a method. Although your patient's use of vitamin C as an analgesic has no scientific basis, there is no problem with her continuing to take it in reasonable doses. Her faith in the method probably causes a placebo effect.

Unfortunately, some patients use potentially harmful methods to relieve pain. Common examples are the ingestion of high doses of alcohol or tranquilizers. These methods most often are used to relieve chronic pain, but they are also used for acute pain. Weaning these patients away from their inappropriate use of potentially destructive chemicals can be quite difficult and usually requires the intervention of a specialist.

SURGICAL APPROACHES

Although nurses have little decision-making responsibility with regard to the use of surgery to control pain, they should have a general understanding of the indications, efficacy, and contraindications for various types of surgical approaches.

Surgery is vastly overrated and overused as a means of eliminating pain. One major pain center reported that it was common to admit patients who had undergone as many as 20–25 operations before entering a pain management program.

Surgical procedures can be effective in relieving pain in cases in which the source of the pain is clearly identified and the diseased tissue can be safely and completely removed (e.g., cholecystic disease or appendicitis). When the source of pain is not obvious or easy to correct, surgery may only add to the patient's suffering. A good example of an ineffective surgical procedure is laminectomy to relieve chronic lower back pain. A large percentage of patients who have laminectomies receive inadequate or no relief from their pain. Even more alarming is the finding that in a significant number of cases, the patients actually experience an increased amount of pain.

Neurosurgical Approaches

Neurosurgical approaches to pain management are generally limited to terminally ill patients who have cancer. Neurosurgery can effectively relieve severe, overwhelming pain that cannot be controlled by less destructive methods. In one procedure, cordotomy, the major pain pathways in the spinal cord are cut. In another procedure, hypophysectomy, the pituitary gland is destroyed. The procedure is usually done through an incision inside the patient's upper lip. The surgeon enters the gland via the nasal cavity and uses microsurgical techniques to destroy the anterior part of the gland. Cryosurgery (freezing) and radiofrequency thermocoagulation are other safe techniques for ablating the pituitary gland.

Cordotomy and hypophysectomy have major undesirable side effects. A common side effect of cordotomy is pronounced weakness of the legs and arms. Another is the inability of some patients to recognize the position of their limbs. Problems may also develop with bowel and bladder control.

Hypophysectomy dramatically alters body chemistry. Appropriate hormone replacement therapy is critically important. Furthermore, if the posterior part of the pituitary gland is accidentally destroyed along with the anterior part, diabetes insipidus will develop.

Three additional problems make these neurosurgical procedures completely unsuitable for any patient not in the final stages of illness:

1. Pain relief is not permanent or predictable. There is absolutely no guarantee that any of these procedures will remove or even lessen the patient's pain.

2. Pain relief does not last. Even in those cases in which the pain is lessened, the relief becomes less and less effective as time goes by.

3. Pain may be made more severe. In some patients, the pain not only returns but is ac-

companied by hyperpathia (intense sensitivity to normal stimuli), causing an explosive pain response.

One pain syndrome, causalgia, responds fairly well to a neurosurgical procedure called sympathectomy. If the condition is detected before irreparable changes take place in the limb, sympathectomy can produce permanent pain relief. This is the only nonterminal condition for which a neurosurgical procedure is indicated for pain relief.

Regional Blocks

Most persons know how effective a nerve block can be in eliminating pain because of their experience with nerve blocks during dental procedures. Nerve blocks (regional blocks) have also been used for years to anesthetize regions of the body during surgery or childbirth. Recently, use of regional blocks to control postoperative pain in a variety of surgical procedures has increased tremendously. The postoperative use of blocks is discussed in more detail in a later chapter.

Because regional blocks generally last only a few hours or days, their usefulness is usually limited to treatment of acute pain. They are used in patients with chronic pain, however, to help determine the sources of pain. For example, a spinal block can be used to determine whether sympathetic or sensory nerves are involved in a pain problem.

Occasionally, regional blocks are made permanent in an attempt to control specific types of pain. In chronic pancreatitis, for example, a temporary nerve block of the celiac ganglion may provide good pain relief. In such a case, pain relief can be provided for several months or more by injecting the ganglion with alcohol to destroy the nerve. Unfortunately, each time a block of this type is repeated, it becomes less effective.

Acupuncture

Although acupunture has been used for more than 2000 years in China, it is only within the last decade that Western medical practitioners have recognized it as an effective means of relieving pain. The scientific basis for acupuncture is the intense stimulation of cutaneous nerve fibers. Although traditional acupuncture relies on precise placement of the needles in "body meridians," modern studies have shown that it is the intensity of the stimulus more than the site of stimulation that determines the degree of pain relief achieved. In fact, needles are not required for the relief of pain. Other sources of intense stimulation, such as electrical stimulation (see TENS section), are equally effective.

BEHAVIORAL INTERVENTIONS

Behavioral methods of pain control are based on the results of research on the cognitive influences on pain (see chapter 2). Some patients (and physicians) doubt that behavior-based techniques can relieve pain. Some patients perceive the suggestion that they use such methods as an indication that the severity of their pain is being questioned. Thus, it is important that nurses establish a trusting relationship with the patient before suggesting a behavioral technique to control pain. Also, they should not try to replace an analgesic with a behavioral method not familiar to the patient. Instead, the behavioral method should be used as an adjunct, at least in the beginning.

Distraction techniques help patients focus on stimuli other than the pain. The pain thus ceases to be the center of attention. It is banished to the periphery of the patient's awareness for various lengths of time. Many patients have learned on their own how to use distraction strategies for pain relief. Common dis-tractions spontaneously used by persons in pain are favorite television shows, visitors, and music.

One myth that interferes with the management of pain is the misconception that any patient who can be distracted must not be having much pain. Regrettably, a patient's ability to use distraction to significantly reduce awareness of pain is often assumed to be proof that the patient's pain is not severe. Health professionals should encourage patients to use this safe and effective way of reducing pain. Instead they discourage patients by disbelieving the pain complaints of any patient who does not act as if the pain is always present. The common response to seeing a patient enjoying a television show or talking with visitors is for the nurse to delay or reduce the patient's next dose of analgesic medication.

Visual Concentration Point and Rhythmic Massage

One behavioral intervention involves the use of a visual focal point and concurrent massaging of skin in a rhythmic, circular manner. This strategy is simple enough that it can be effectively used for either mild or very severe pain. Patients with mild pain do not need anything more complex; those with severe pain cannot cope with complex maneuvers. (Those with severe pain normally use this technique as an adjunct to other pain control techniques.)

A major asset of this strategy is that it can be taught to highly anxious patients facing imminent painful procedures. It quickly gives the patients some sense of control over what they are experiencing. The circular massage can be started by the nurse and transferred to the patient.

Breathing Techniques

Slow, rhythmic breathing. The patient takes a cleansing breath at the beginning and the end of each session. The rate of breathing is approximately 6–9 breaths/min. Inhalation should be controlled so that it is slow and even, and breath-holding should be avoided. Exhalation is slow and passive. The patient can breathe through the nose or the mouth. Several motions can be included with the breathing to increase the complexity of this technique (e.g., raising and lowering a finger or arm in rhythm with the breathing). This technique can be effective for mild or moderate pain. A more active method, such as the "he-who" breathing technique described in the next section, is usually needed for severe pain.

He-who breathing. The patient whispers "he" on exhalation, then inhales, then whispers "who" on exhalation. No sound is used during inhalation. This he-who rhythm is repeated over and over. The rate begins slowly and increases as the pain becomes more intense. Breathing must be shallow to avoid hyperventilation. Both a focal point and rhythmic massage can be added to increase the effectiveness of this technique.

Pant-blow rhythmic breathing. The patient uses a series of five breaths: four panting breaths followed by a blowing breath. The rate of this rhythmic breathing begins slowly and increases as pain becomes more intense. The rate should not exceed 60 breaths/min. Because breathing rapidly through the nose is difficult, the patient is advised to breathe through the mouth.

Other Techniques

Sing and tap. Silently mouthing words to a song while keeping time by tapping a finger or foot is an effective method for providing a distraction from pain. The speed of the tapping can be accelerated as the intensity of the pain increases. The technique starts and ends with a cleansing breath. Patients should also be instructed to stop and take a cleansing breath at any point they feel the need for one. This procedure can easily be taught to older children as well as to adults.

Describing a series of pictures. The patient describes to another person a group of pictures that the patient finds interesting.

Auditory stimulation via earphones. Music selected by the patient is listened to through earphones. Mental images and keeping rhythm can be added for enhanced distraction.

Humor. Books, magazines, movies, and so forth that particularly appeal to the patient can be used to provide distraction from pain for several hours at a time.

HYPNOTHERAPY

Hypnosis

Hypnosis can be defined as a state of alertness characterized by attentive, receptive, focal concentration with diminished peripheral awareness (Debetz, 1981). It has been used for many years to control pain and relax muscles and even to facilitate healing. Hypnotic techniques used to control pain vary, but generally include some of the following (Wakeman & Kaplan, 1978):

- Blocking awareness of the pain

- Substituting another feeling (such as pressure) for the pain

- Moving the pain to a smaller or less significant area of the body

- Changing the meaning of the pain so that it is less important

- Distorting time

- In extreme cases, dissociating the body from the patient's awareness

Guided Imagery

Another hypnotherapy technique used for pain control is guided imagery. Patients are taught to use their imagination to develop mental images that decrease the intensity of pain or become a pleasant or painless substitute for pain. Guided imagery conducted by patients on their own is similar to some forms of self-hypnosis. It is hoped that the pain relief provided will last as long as several hours after the use of imagery. Useful side effects are muscle relaxation and a decrease in anxiety, which can help patients who are having problems falling asleep.

RELAXATION TECHNIQUES

As has been mentioned several times, the perception of pain can be increased by increased stress or emotional tension. Most health care professionals think that stress and muscle tension are significant factors in prolonging chronic pain. Relaxation is also used as one aspect of pain relief for a variety of acute pain conditions (e.g., childbirth).

Use of relaxation techniques by a patient with pain can do the following (McCaffery, 1979):

● Reduce the effects of stress

● Decrease acute anxiety

● Act as a distraction from pain

● Alleviate skeletal muscle tension or contraction that is creating potentially painful stimuli

● Combat fatigue and facilitate going to sleep

● Enhance the effectiveness of other pain relief measures

Although relaxation techniques can be beneficial for patients with pain, relaxation does not always relieve pain and sometimes even exacerbates it. This may be due to an increased awareness of the pain. When used as the only noninvasive method of pain relief during childbirth, for instance, the relaxation technique was not effective in many instances. On the other hand, use of relaxation techniques has successfully relieved several types of acute pain of short duration (e.g., tension headache and postoperative pain).

Few persons, including health care professionals, have an accurate understanding of what constitutes relaxation. Many assume that lying on the couch in front of the television set is relaxation. Others equate relaxation with reading a book or more vigorous activities such as playing tennis or weeding the garden. Unfortunately, in all these situations, the participant may still maintain physiological and psychological states characteristic of chronic stress. Even during sleep, muscle tension may be maintained at high levels. Thus, persons often think they are relaxed when they are not.

Many ways can be used to elicit the relaxation response. Four basic elements are thought to be necessary components of an effective relaxation technique.

1. Quiet environment

2. Comfortable position

3. Mental device (e.g., mantra, phrases, heartbeat, visual foci)

4. Passive attitude (person's awareness centered on feelings of relaxation, sending away distracting worries, noises, and so forth)

In-depth discussions of relaxation techniques are available in a variety of texts, including McCaffery's. Nurses interested in using this technique personally or in the clinical setting should consult these other resources.

BIOFEEDBACK

Many physiological functions (e.g., blood pressure and pulse rate) depend on the autonomic nervous system. Biofeedback is a technique in which a person is made aware of changes in bodily functions, with the aim of eventually controlling the functions to advantage (autoregulation). It has been used in the management of pain due to tension headaches, migraines, and lower back disorders. No well-controlled studies have been performed to prove the effectiveness of biofeedback. Some specialists think the benefit seen with this method is probably due to distraction, suggestion, relaxation, and a sense of control over the pain (Melzack, Taenzer, Feldman, & Kinch, 1981). It has not been any more effective for tension headaches than relaxation.

SKIN STIMULATION

Persons instinctively use two skin-stimulation techniques to control pain (particularly sudden, acute pain such as that caused by hitting an elbow against a sharp object). These techniques are pressure and massage. By stimulating a variety of skin receptors in the area surrounding the injured area, they partially close the spinal gate to pain impulses from that area.

Skin stimulation can relieve different types of pain. However, predicting the particular types of stimulation that will provide the greatest pain relief for each patient is difficult. A trial-and-error approach is usually required.

Pressure

Firm pressure should be applied with hands or a firm object (e.g., tennis ball, sandbag) near the painful area or with a finger or palm on the appropriate acupuncture site or trigger point.

Massage

Massage of the painful area or a nearby region can help reduce pain. Because the amount of pressure required is variable, it used should be regulated by the patient.

Vibration

Vibration can be quite effective in reducing pain. Vibration devices include hand-held electric vibrators, slipper-type vibrators for the feet, and vibrating pads.

Chemical Skin Stimulants

Another method of stimulating the skin is the application of over-the-counter lotions, ointments, gels, and liniments claimed to relieve sore muscles, backs, and joints. Application of these substances to the skin covering the painful area actually can be quite effective for mild to moderate muscle, bone, and joint discomfort. The underlying mechanisms are probably a combination of distraction, stimulation of multiple skin sensors, and some placebo effect.

These chemical skin stimulants can also be classified as counterirritants. The use of irritating substances on the skin to reduce pain is a common practice in primitive cultures and folk remedies. Generally, these compounds are quite safe and amazingly effective and inexpensive.

TRANSCUTANEOUS ELECTRICAL NERVE STIMULATION

All nerves within approximately 4 cm below the surface of the skin can be stimulated by placing electrodes on the skin surface. The most widely used TENS method uses a small, battery-powered electronic pulse generator about the size of a pack of cigarettes. The patient usually feels a buzzing, tingling, or vibrating sensation, and the intensity and quality of skin stimulation can be adjusted by the patient.

The precise mechanism by which nerve stimulation relieves pain is not clear. According to the gate theory, TENS stimulates the large-diameter cutaneous nerve fibers, closing the gate in the spinal cord to transmission of pain impulses to the thalamus. It appears to do this by raising the firing threshold of the cells in the spinal cord, directly inhibiting them from responding to painful stimuli. Also, the inhibitory system within the brainstem appears to be activated, further raising the firing threshold in the cells in the spinal cord. Many different explanations have been put forward by researchers to explain the analgesia created by TENS. For example, TENS may increase the production of the body's own opioid analgesic: endorphins. Another probable benefit of TENS is that it increases the blood flow to the area of stimulation.

A prescription form a physician is required to begin TENS therapy. The effectiveness of the therapy depends on a number of factors: placement, intensity, duration, and frequency. Appropriate placement of the electrodes largely depends on the site of the pain, but recommendations for placement also vary among the many manufacturers of TENS units. Manufacturers' charts for placement of the electrodes should always be consulted. Most often the electrodes are placed over or near the painful site. They can also be placed over the nerve that innervates the painful area.

Intensity is usually started at a moderate level, because mild stimulation may be simply annoying. The current can be raised to a level that may cause muscle contraction, but this degree of stimulation is usually not necessary and may result in muscle soreness. Sometimes only vigorous stimulation is effective, but not all patients can tolerate this intensity. The patient should be the ultimate guide as to what stimulation level is effective in relieving pain.

Stimulation can be done either continuously or intermittently. The duration of intermittent stimulation commonly is 10–30 min. If possible, the frequency should be determined by how long pain relief continues after the cessation of stimulation. Patients who experience pain relief only during the actual cutaneous stimulation can use portable TENS units on a continuous basis.

The most common use for TENS is treatment of chronic pain in adults, but it has also been tried in a broad range of acute pain situations, including postoperatively. It is most effective when the pain is localized in a small area. When TENS is the sole method used to relieve pain, about half of all patients receive significant relief, but this rate declines to about 30–35% after 1 year. If TENS is used as part of a comprehensive pain management program, the success rate is about 65–70% initially, declining to about 50% after 1 year.

Skin irritation sometimes occurs with TENS therapy, but it disappears when the stimulation is stopped. Patients with cardiac pacemakers cannot use this therapy. Overall, TENS is a safe and moderately effective means of reducing pain. It is clearly most effective when used in conjunction with other pain management techniques.

HEAT AND COLD

Pain can be reduced by the application of both heat and cold. Sometimes it is difficult to predict which will be most effective. For example, some persons with back pain find that the application of heat makes the pain worse. Others find that heat is useful in reducing both muscle spasms and pain in the back. The physiological effects of heat and cold differ:

● An inflammatory response may be exacerbated by applications of heat and decreased by applications of cold.

● Blood flow is increased by applications of heat and reduced by applications of cold.

● Edema may be increased by the application of heat and decreased by the application of cold.

● Stiffness in rheumatoid conditions is decreased by applications of heat and increased by applications of cold.

External Analgesics

A multitude of over-the-counter lotions, ointments, gels, and liniments are said to reduce pain. Those containing menthol and methyl salicylate have been superior to a placebo in a number of studies. The most common use of the menthol products is for joint and muscle pain.

Counterirritants

Using counterirritants to relieve pain is a common practice in primitive cultures and is still the principle underlying many home remedies used today. Deep-heat salves, menthol skin ointments, ice packs, hot water bottles, and vigorous massage are all examples of familiar counterirritants. Pain relief may persist for hours after the intervention is stopped. Although the underlying mechanism of pain relief is not known, it is probably similar to that which occurs in TENS. Regardless, counterirritants can be a safe and inexpensive method to relieve mild pain and an adjunct to other methods for moderate or severe pain.

SUMMARY

A wide range of treatments are used to relieve pain. These include drugs, surgical interventions, behavioral interventions, hypnotherapy, relaxation techniques, biofeedback, skin stimulation, TENS, and use of heat and cold. The following chapters examine pain treatments in more detail and in relationship to the specific types of pain being treated.

EXAM QUESTIONS

Chapter 5

Questions 24–30

24. What guideline should be followed to determine the number of pain-relief measures used to manage pain?

    a. Only one pain-relief method should be used at a time.
    b. At least three pain-relief measures should be alternated.
    c. Only nonopioid analgesics should be used with other methods.
    d. A variety of pain-relief measures should be used.

25. In regard to the timing of administration of medication, what guideline should nurses use?

    a. Use pain relief measures sooner rather than later.
    b. Wait until the patient cannot stand the pain any longer.
    c. Avoid early administration in order to decrease the possibility of addiction.
    d. Give only opioid measures later and others sooner.

26. What is an invasive technique sometimes used to control pain in terminally ill patients with cancer?

    a. Laminectomy
    b. Cordotomy
    c. TENS
    d. Sympathectomy

27. What is the physiological effect of cold?

    a. Increased inflammatory response
    b. Increased blood flow
    c. Decreased bleeding
    d. Increased edema

28. What does applications of heat decrease in rheumatoid conditions?

    a. Inflammatory response
    b. Edema
    c. Stiffness
    d. Blood flow

29. What noninvasive pain control measure uses a battery-powered electronic pulse generator to provide stimulation to the skin surface?

    a. Acupressure or acupuncture
    b. Counterirritants
    c. Lumbar epidural blocks
    d. TENS

30. What is a disadvantage of using cordotomy to relieve pain?

    a. It can cause pronounced weakness in the arms and legs.
    b. Diabetes insipidus is a frequent side effect.
    c. The patient will need hormone replacement therapy.
    d. Speech problems often develop after the procedure.

CHAPTER 6

PHARMACOLOGICAL CONTROL OF PAIN: GENERAL GUIDELINES

CHAPTER OBJECTIVE

After studying this chapter, the reader will be able to describe the mechanisms, durations, onsets, and major side effects of analgesics and specify dosages equianalgesic to morphine.

LEARNING OBJECTIVES

After studying this chapter, the reader will be able to

1. Specify the overriding fear that is the reason health care professionals do not take advantage of available analgesics.

2. Recognize the major mechanism by which nonsteroidal antiinflammatory drugs reduce pain.

3. Indicate the major side effects of opioid analgesics.

4. Describe how the route of administration influences the action of an analgesic.

5. Specify the dose of intramuscular meperidine that is equianalgesic to 10 mg of intramuscular morphine.

6. Indicate the duration and onset of action of 10 mg of morphine given intramuscularly.

INTRODUCTION

Powerful and sophisticated treatments are available for the treatment of pain. Nevertheless, pain continues to be a major problem (Grossman, Sheidler, Swedeen, Mucenski, & Piantadosi, 1990; Lander, 1990; Roark, 1991; Slack & Faut-Callahan, 1991). Some of the reasons for this deplorable situation have been mentioned in previous chapters: the inadequate assessment of pain and common myths about pain behaviors that interfere with the recognition and treatment of pain. This chapter discusses the detrimental effects of undertreatment and takes a closer look at drugs used to treat pain.

Pain Can Kill

Pain is not just a regrettable but relatively harmless side effect of disease, injury, treatments, and certain normal conditions (e.g., childbirth). Severe pain is a life-threatening condition. Treatment of this condition should be approached with same degree of resolve as that used for all other threats to a patient's life.

Too many physicians and nurses, however, continue to view pain as a nuisance, and they give it only grudging attention. Pain is often low on the list of treatment priorities for a seriously ill patient. Of much higher priority are treatments recognized as important to survival: blood transfusions, antibiotics, chemotherapy, and so forth. Severe pain is usually not recognized as a threat to the patient's ultimate survival.

Pain control is also viewed as the intended outcome of adequately treating the underlying disease or injury. The reasoning is that too much time should not be spent on controlling the patient's pain because pain will cease to be a problem once the underlying disorder is treated.

Uncontrolled pain can undercut efforts to treat the patient's disease. Severe pain and stress can inhibit immune function (Keller, Weiss, Schleifer, Miller, & Stein, 1981) and enhance tumor growth (Sklar & Anisman, 1979) in laboratory animals. In a recent editorial in *Pain*, Liebeskind (1991) discusses the findings of new research that showed the adverse effects of pain in laboratory animals and the effectiveness of analgesics in preventing these adverse effects. He states, "These results . . . suggest it is not only safe to use analgesic drugs for controlling cancer pain in man, it may be unsafe not to." He goes on to describe his own research, which shows that even a single exposure to stress significantly increases the metastatic spread of cancer in laboratory mice. A similar result was observed when rats underwent standard laparotomy under anesthesia. In humans, severe acute pain associated with surgery or trauma can cause profound pathophysiological changes. Recent clinical studies (Multgren, 1990) indicate that effective pain management can decrease both morbidity and mortality.

It is not clear whether it is the pain itself or the stress reaction caused by it that reduces the immune response and speeds the growth of tumors. What is clear is that pain of sufficient intensity poses a serious threat to the patient. As the pain researcher Melzack (1988) noted: "Pain can . . . have a major impact on morbidity and mortality; . . . it can mean the difference between life and death."

EFFECTIVENESS OF ANALGESICS

The development of highly purified natural and synthetic analgesics during the past 50 years has provided physicians with a large array of safe compounds to control pain of all intensities. Despite the availability of these powerful drugs, however, uncontrolled pain continues to be commonplace.

For many years, part of the problem was a lack of adequate information about the analgesics available. Few or no data were available to explain how the various analgesics worked, how well they were absorbed by the body, how long they were active in the body, or even how much analgesia each drug could provide. Although this gap has been filled for nearly a decade now, the overall effectiveness of analgesic therapy has not improved significantly.

What, then, are the problems that interfere with the effective use of analgesics? An early study conducted in two teaching hospitals showed that 73% of patients having pain continued to have pain of moderate to severe intensity despite treatment with analgesics (Marks & Sachar, 1973). The reasons physicians and nurses did not use available analgesics to the full advantage of these drugs were as follows:

1. Exaggerated fears of side effects (e.g., drowsiness, urinary retention, constipation, and respiratory depression)

2. An almost irrational fear that patients would become addicted

3. A curious belief among house officers that very low doses of opioids were effective against severe pain and that higher doses would provide no added relief

The additive effects of these misconceptions on patient care were pronounced:

> [Analgesic] drugs are given in doses that are often inadequate, at time intervals that are often too long, according to a regimen [prn], that requires the patient to wait out the time interval, no matter how severe the pain. Even the inadequate amounts of opioids ordered may not in fact be received by the patient. The prn regimen, by placing the onus on the patient to request the drug, introduces considerations other than whether or not he is in pain. Patients may be inhibited by a desire to please the medical staff and not be a nuisance. Those who do decide to ask for pain relief must keep track of both the time and the drug schedule and have the strength and endurance to summon a nurse. . . . The extent to which nurses share the common concerns about addiction may influence their readiness to respond. Thus, in practice, the average daily dose of opioids received is even smaller than the amounts ordered and not correlated with the degree of persistent pain. (Marks & Sachar, 1973)

Part of the problem has also been that health care professionals were not held responsible for providing adequate pain relief. This is likely to change because of the ground-breaking decision of a jury in North Carolina. The jury found a nursing home and its nursing staff guilty of negligence in failing to provide a patient with adequate pain medication. The nursing home was ordered to pay the patient's estate $15 million. This is the type of case pain experts have been waiting for. Finally, health care professionals will be held legally responsible for providing adequate pain relief to their patients.

According to an article in the *Los Angeles Times* (Roark, 1991), this case exposed a number of erroneous myths and misguided nursing practices that prevented a terminally ill cancer patient from receiving adequate pain medication. The patient involved had prostatic cancer with multiple bone metastases that caused excruciating pain.

The nursing supervisor at the home considered herself the authority on how much pain the cancer patient, Mr. James, was experiencing and how much pain he should be able to tolerate. She testified during the trial about her husband's experience with cancer (colostomy, thoracotomy, and abdominal surgery). She told how during all this her husband never asked for morphine, nor would she have given it to him. She also related how she herself had had a mastectomy for breast cancer. After surgery she had not needed morphine. "I had my surgery on a Friday; on Sunday I took two Tylenol," she testified.

Her testimony in court also showed that she misunderstood the concepts of addiction, tolerance, and the proper use of opioids in the treatment of chronic, progressive pain in the terminally ill. She testified how she had "warned [the patient] of the dangers [of the high dose of morphine he had been taking at the hospital] that he could become addicted, that he could become so tolerant to the medication that it would stop working altogether."

Under her direction, the nursing staff radically reduced the patient's pain medication (the order had been medication every 4 hr as needed for pain). "The nursing records showed [the patient] was denied six, seven, sometimes eight doses a day. In all, the experts calculated, he had gone from 240 doses of morphine in January to only 41 in February."

Unfortunately, this case is not an isolated incident. Thousands of patients in the United States are enduring unnecessary pain because of misguided professionals. Only through the dissemination of better information about pain management, and greater demands for professional accountability, will the number of patients with uncontrolled pain be reduced.

The information in this textbook can be used to effect an overall improvement in the manner in which analgesics are administered in the health care setting. Making changes of this magnitude requires a high level of commitment. Persistence and even courage will be needed to encourage physicians to write better orders for analgesics and nurses to administer the drugs more effectively. Nurses' efforts on behalf of pain patients may not be appreciated by some physicians and colleagues. However, improving the level of pain relief given to hundreds of patients can be among the most important contributions a nurse can make.

DIFFERENCES BETWEEN NONOPIOID AND OPIOID ANALGESICS

Analgesics are commonly defined as drugs that reduce the intensity of pain without causing loss of consciousness. They can be separated into two main categories: nonopioid and opioid.

Nonopioid Analgesics

Each day over-the-counter nonopioid analgesics are used by millions for the treatment of a variety of painful conditions. In addition to their ability to reduce pain, many nonopioid analgesics have other desirable effects: reduction of inflammation, fever, and formation of blood clots.

Nonopioid analgesics vary in their analgesic potency as well as in their antiinflammatory and antipyretic effectiveness. The most widely used nonopioid drug for the past century has been aspirin (acetylsalicylic acid). In recent years, however, both acetaminophen (e.g., Tylenol) and ibuprofen (e.g., Advil or Motrin) have been gaining popularity as over-the-counter pain remedies.

Nonopioids are generally given orally and are most useful in the treatment of mild to moderate pain, or as an adjunct to opioid analgesics. Unlike opioid analgesics, nonopioids do not cause sedation and are not addictive. The major drawback of nonopioid analgesics is that they have a therapeutic ceiling or limit to their analgesic potency. Doses greater than these therapeutic limits do not provide additional analgesia, only additional side effects.

Most of the nonopioid drugs appear to act directly on injured tissues, not on peripheral nerves or in the central nervous system. The therapeutic effect is most likely due to the ability to block the synthesis of prostaglandins, powerful hormones that trigger an inflammatory reaction in injured tissues. Because their potent inhibition of prostaglandins, nonopioid analgesics are referred to as NSAIDs. They are often used to treat pain due to inflammation caused by disease or injury (e.g., arthritis, muscle injuries).

Side effects are common with nonopioid analgesics, but they are usually minor. Gastrointestinal effects and increased bleeding are seen most often with increasing doses. Every nurse should be familiar with the major side effects and contraindications for each type of analgesic. Problems associated with prolonged, frequent use of analgesics are discussed in chapter 7.

Opioid Analgesics

Greek and Roman physicians used preparations containing the narcotic opium to relieve arthritic pain, chest pain, and prolonged coughing spells. The term *opiates* was derived from the Greek word for poppy juice, the original source of opium. The term *morphine* was derived from Morpheus, the name of the Greek god of sleep. Both natural and synthetic opioid analgesics are referred to as opiates or as morphine and its cogeners.

Opioid analgesics can be subcategorized in a number of ways. This text classifies them as either weak analgesics (for mild to moderate pain) or potent analgesics (for moderate to severe pain) on the basis of their analgesic potency. Weak opioid analgesics include codeine, propoxyphene, and oxycodone. Potent opioid analgesics include morphine, hydromorphone, and methadone. The term *potency* refers to the intrinsic analgesic properties of a drug; the potency of morphine is used as the standard.

Unlike the nonopioid analgesics, which act directly on injured tissues, opioid analgesics exert their effects on the opiate receptors in the central nervous system. Opioids can also be categorized according to the manner in which they interact with opiate receptors. Opioids classified as agonists bind to opiate receptors. Morphine is the prototypical agonist drug. Opioids classified as agonist-antagonists, on the other hand, reverse or block the effects of morphine. Agonist-antagonists such as pentazocine (Talwin) and butorphanol (Stadol), exert an analgesic effect while blocking the effect of morphine. The antagonist drug naloxone is unique in that it is a pure antagonist with no analgesic effect. The only use for naloxone is to reverse the effects of excessive doses of opioid agonists such as morphine.

To avoid inadvertently giving agonists and antagonists to the same patient, nurses should always be familiar with the category of each analgesic they administer. When a patient who is regularly receiving an agonist-antagonist (e.g., pentazocine) is given a dose of an agonist (e.g., morphine), the antagonist properties of the first drug will be blocked by the analgesic effect of the agonist.

It is currently thought that all opioid analgesics produce their analgesic effects by binding to discrete opiate receptors in the peripheral and central nervous systems. The major side effects associated with opioid analgesics are a decrease in alertness and, when used for long period, tolerance, physical dependence, and potential addiction.

GUIDELINES FOR ADMINISTERING ANALGESICS

The information in the next section is presented in a question-and-answer format. The questions are ones often asked by nurses who are learning more about how to administer analgesics so that patients have maximum pain relief without unnecessary side effects (Table 6-1). Much of this information has been learned from nurses, pharmacologists, psychologists, and physicians who are specialists in the treatment of pain. These guidelines are intended for use with terminally ill patients who have acute pain. The special guidelines that should be followed when working with patients with chronic pain are presented in a later chapter.

Q: How does the route of administration affect a drug's activity?

A: Opioid analgesics can be administered by a wide variety of routes: oral, subcutaneous, sublingual, intramuscular, intravenous, transdermal, intrathecal, epidural, and intraventricular. Not all opioids are suitable for all routes of administration, however. Nonopioid analgesics are almost always given by the oral route.

TABLE 6-1
Information Needed for Proper Administration of Analgesics

Information the Nurse Should Have About the Patient

- How much pain is the patient currently experiencing?
- Where is the pain located, and what are its characteristics?
- What medication has the patient taken previously for this pain and how well did it (they) work? When was the last dose administered?
- What is the health team's goal for pain management in this patient, and does the patient understand the goal?
- What is the patient's goal for pain relief, and is it consistent with the health team's plan?

Information the Nurse Should Have About the Prescibed Analgesics

- What are the relative potencies or doses of the prescribed medications?
- How rapid is the onset of analgesia, and what is the average duration of analgesia?
- Could analgesics be combined to improve the patient's pain control?
- Are there other pain relief interventions that could be used in combination with an analgesic?

The route of administration influences a drug's action in a number of predictable ways. Generally speaking, administration of drugs by mouth or by rectum slows the drugs' onset of action and prolongs the duration of action. Parenteral administration, on the other hand, speeds the onset and shortens the duration.

The most rapid onset of action is achieved with intravenous administration; the duration of action is also the shortest. When the goal is to relieve a patient's pain as quickly as possible, the intravenous route of administration should be selected. When the goal is to prolong a drug's analgesic effect, the oral route is preferable.

Q: Are all analgesics similar in the duration of their analgesic effects?

A: Just as opioids vary in how quickly they start providing pain relief, they also vary in how long the pain relief lasts. In general, the faster the onset is, the shorter the duration of analgesia.

The most common error made by physicians when ordering analgesics is assuming that a drug provides pain relief far longer than the drug actually does. It is not uncommon for physicians to think that meperidine (Demerol) provides analgesia for 3–4 hr, when, in fact, meperidine's analgesic effect usually begins to disappear (or totally disappears) within 2.5 hr. (This is particularly true with the first or second dose.)

Unnecessary pain can be avoided if nurses become more knowledgeable about the expected duration of analgesia produced by each of the opioids they administer (Table 6-2). This way inadequate orders for analgesics can be recognized as soon as the orders are written rather than be discovered after the prescribed doses fail to relieve a patient's pain.

TABLE 6-2

Equianalgesic Doses of Narcotic Analgesics for Moderate to Severe Pain

Analgesic Medication	Equianalgesic Doses PO (mg)	Equianalgesic Doses IM (mg)	Equivalent Dose of IM Morphine (mg)	Onset PO (minutes)	Onset IM (minutes)	Peak Effect (minutes)	Duration (hours)
Meperidine	300	75	10	60–90	30–60	50–99	3
Hydromorphone	7.5	1.5	10	30–45	15–30	60	2–3
Levorphanol	4.0	2.0	10	30–60	—	120	4–7
Dolophine	20	10	10	30–60	30–45	—	4–5
Morphine	60	—	10	30–60	30–45	—	4–7
Oxymorphine	10 mg rectally		10	—	NA	120	4–6
Percodan or Percocet	6 tabs	—	10	10–15	NA	45	3–6
Butorphanol	—	2	10	—	rapid	30	2.5–3.5
Nalbuphine	—	10	10	30–60	30–45	120	3–4
Pentazocine	120	60	10	30–60	30–45	120	3–4
Fentanyl	—	0.2	10	—	rapid	—	—

Note: PO = orally, IM = intramuscularly, NA = not applicable.

For example, if an order says, "Meperidine 75–100 mg intramuscularly every 4 hr as needed for pain," the nurse can immediately discuss the order with the physician. Most physicians will be surprised to learn that the analgesic effect of meperidine is so short. Open-minded ones will switch to another medication or shorten the interval between doses of meperidine. Those who are not as open-minded will need to be called repeatedly by the nurse and told that their patients are in pain again.

Q: What does the term *relative potency* mean? Do I need to pay attention to it? (It sounds like something only a pharmacist or physician needs to know.)

A: Any time a nurse selects an analgesic from a list of two or more drugs, he or she needs to know about the relative potency of the drugs listed. Most nurses probably already have a "gut feeling" for the relative potencies of the various analgesics. That is, they have a general idea about which analgesics are stronger and which are weaker. Relative potency is just a more precise measure of a drug's ability to reduce pain. Thus, the relative potency of each analgesic drug is its strength compared with a 10-mg dose of intramuscular morphine. For example, Table 7-5 in chapter 7 shows that 130 mg of oral codeine is required to provide analgesia equal to that provided by 10 mg of morphine given intramuscularly or intravenously. This indicates that parenteral morphine is 13 times more potent than oral codeine.

How can relative potency information be used in clinical practice? When called on to select an analgesic from a list of several drugs ordered for a particular patient, the nurse can use information about the relative potencies of these drugs to make a choice. Say, for example, a patient is complaining of moderately severe pain. A check of the patient's orders reveals a list of analgesics with a range of potencies, from 30 mg of oral codeine up to 75 mg of intramuscular meperidine. The nurse could follow a gut feeling and choose meperidine. Or, he or she could make a more informed selection by using the information in Table 7-5. The second approach greatly increases the likelihood that the drug ultimately administered will adequately relieve the patient's pain without producing excessive side effects.

The most important time to use relative potency data, however, is when patients are being switched from one form of a drug to another form. Usually this means that a patient who has been receiving parenteral opioids for pain control is being switched to an oral analgesic so that he or she can be discharged. Problems usually arise because the physician guesses about how many milligrams of an oral opioid are required to equal the parenteral analgesic and makes the usual mistake of overestimating the potency of the oral form of the opioid.

However, it is not difficult to figure out how much oral opioid is equal to the intramuscular or intravenous dose the patient has been receiving. All that is needed is a look at a relative potency chart. For example, a patient has been receiving 10 mg of morphine intramuscularly. Table 6-2 shows that 60 mg of morphine given orally is equal (equianalgesic) to 10 mg of morphine given intramuscularly or intravenously. Therefore, the potency of oral morphine is only one sixth the potency of parenteral morphine.

Q: I have seen charts showing how long after an opioid is administered peak analgesia occurs. Is it important to know this information?

A: It can be very useful. Suppose a nurse administers 10 mg of morphine intramuscularly to a patient for pain. Two hours later, the patient says that the pain has not decreased very much. At that point, the nurse has two alternatives: (1) wait and see if the patient's pain decreases further during the next 1–2 hr (intramuscular morphine can provide analgesia for up to 6 hr) or (2) contact the patient's physician right away to get additional orders for analgesics.

Nurses who are aware that intramuscular morphine provides peak analgesia 2 hr after administration will know that the patient is currently experiencing maximum pain relief. They would contact the physician as soon as possible, as it is obvious that the patient is not going to become more comfortable without additional morphine. It would be cruel to delay another 2 hr before giving the patient more analgesia.

Q: Are there major differences in the half-lives of opioid analgesics? If so, what significance does it have for controlling pain?

A: A drug's half-life is the time it takes for half of the absorbed dose to be metabolized and eliminated from the body. This information indicates how long a drug is likely to remain in a patient's system. Also, depending on the site of metabolism, the half-life of some drugs will be prolonged in patients with impaired kidney or liver function.

Most drugs do not accumulate to higher and higher levels in the bloodstream of patients with normal kidney and liver function. Less than half of the active drug remains in the body when subsequent doses are given. However, when a drug with a long half-life is repeatedly administered before more than half the previous dose is metabolized, the drug will accumulate in the patient's blood. Eventually, amount of the drug in the blood will increase to a toxic level.

Methadone is one opioid analgesic that is slowly eliminated from the body. It has a half-life of 15–30 hr. Despite this prolonged half-life, methadone must be given every 4–6 hr (in the early stages of treatment), because the duration of the analgesia it provides is only 4–6 hr.

After a patient has received methadone every 4 hr for several days, the drug will have accumulated in the blood. This is why signs and symptoms of a drug overdose (e.g., excessive sedation, confusion, and respiratory depression) often appear days after routine doses of methadone have been started. Contrary to what might be expected, the solution to this dilemma is not to reduce the dose of methadone. Rather, it is better to increase the interval between doses. The level of methadone in the blood will remain high enough to maintain the patient's comfort even when doses are given every 8–12 hrs. This ability of methadone to maintain adequately high levels of analgesia with infrequent doses is one reason it is used to treat pain caused by cancer. Patients get steady pain control with less fluctuation in sedation and only need to take a few doses each day.

Special care is needed to avoid overmedicating patients when drugs with long half-lives are used. In cases of serious overmedication with such a drug, it takes days for the side effects (e.g., excessive sedation, depressed respirations) to begin disappearing. With short-acting opioids, on the other hand, the signs and symptoms of overdose resolve in just a few hours.

Q: With regards to administering analgesic medications to patients, other than noting the dose, route, and so forth in the chart, what should I be writing in my nursing notes?

A: Each patient's response to a given dose of analgesic is unpredictable. This is particularly true with opioids. Furthermore, factors such as previous exposure to opioids, the intensity of the pain, body weight, kidney function, and age affect how much pain relief the patient experiences and how many side effects occur. In addition, the same patient may vary tremendously in his or her response to the same dose of the same analgesic from injection to injection. Exactly why this occurs is not known.

Thus, it is important that the nursing notes fully reflect the patient's situation before and after administration of analgesics. How severe was the pain at the time the drug was administered? How much pain relief did the patient experience? Did the pain return before the next dose of analgesic could be given? Did any untoward side effects (e.g., nausea and vomiting, constipation, urinary retention, lethargy) occur? At least once per shift, a description of the patient's pain (e.g., location, intensity) should be added to the patient's chart (see the guidelines provided in the chapter on pain assessment). This is the evaluation step in the nursing process in caring for patients in pain. It allows the nurse to take the information about the patient's response and use it in revising the care plan.

Q: What is patient-controlled analgesia (PCA) and does it provide improved comfort for the patient?

A: Technology now provides a way for patients to safely self-administer intravenous opioids for acute or chronic pain by using a special pump. The general procedure for PCA is to load the pump with an opioid diluted in a small amount of intravenous solution. The pump can then be set to deliver a specified amount of opioid each time the patient presses a button. A "lockout" period is also set to avoid overmedication. During this lockout period, the patient cannot self-administer additional doses. A common lockout period is 10 min.

When used properly, PCA is highly effective for treating a wide variety of painful conditions. Several factors account for this. For one thing, no delay occurs between the patient's request for additional pain medication and the actual administration of the medication. Furthermore, PCA provides patients with greater control over their pain. They can decide when and how much additional medication is needed. Research has shown that persons who can exert some control over their pain experience less pain. Thus, it is likely that the increased control offered by PCA contributes to its improved analgesic effect. It is also likely that patients who use PCA experience less anxiety, as they do not have to convince a nurse that they need another dose of analgesic or that the previous doses were not strong enough. Less anxiety also contributes to better pain control.

The answer to the next question provides an additional explanation as to why PCA works so well in controlling pain.

Q: Should patients with acute pain be encouraged to wait as long as possible before requesting or self-administering additional pain medication?

A: Many health care professionals cling to the notion that analgesic medications should be kept to a minimum in order to avoid troublesome side effects and complications. Clinical experience has shown, however, that when pain is relieved in its beginning stages, before it has made the patient tense, the relief can be achieved more rapidly and completely. Nevertheless, many a health care professional continues to advise patients to wait for additional pain medication until they are sure they really "need it."

Figure 6-1 shows the pattern of pain relief seen when patients receive analgesics after pain has become substantial. The shaded area represents uncontrolled pain; the unshaded area represents controlled pain (i.e., the pain has been relieved). The jagged line on the graph represents the patient's level of analgesia. The deep fluctuations in this line indicate that the patient is going from a high level of analgesia (and probably sedation) to very low levels with little or no pain control.

Figure 6-2 shows the pattern when additional analgesics are given when the analgesia starts wearing off and before the patient is in pain. At no time is the pain poorly controlled. The fluctuations in the levels of analgesia are also less extreme, so the patient is not going back and forth from oversedation to no sedation.

Patients using PCA are most likely to achieve this consistent level of pain relief. This requires, of course, that they have been instructed to self-administer additional doses of analgesic when their comfort is beginning to decrease rather than waiting until the pain has returned.

Q: Do I need to know the mechanism of action for every analgesic medication?

A: In several situations, it is useful to know how various analgesics work. For example, nurses who are involved in teaching patients how to take pain medications properly should be aware that use of NSAIDs, such as Motrin, should not be restricted to periods of pain if the medications are being prescribed to reduce inflammation (e.g., for bursitis, or tendinitis). A steady blood level of the drug is needed for days or even weeks in order to adequately reduce inflammation. Patients are likely to stop taking the medication once the pain begins to disappear unless they have been advised to keep taking the drug regularly for the entire time indicated by the physician. (The patient can be told that the inflam-

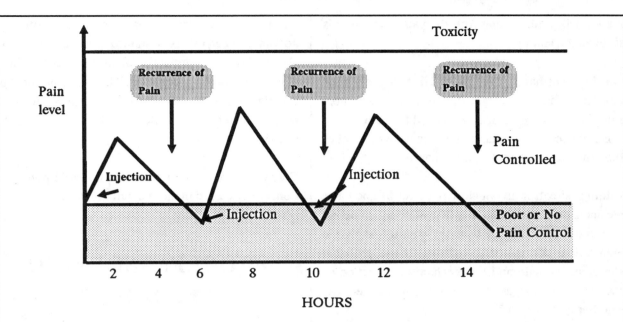

Toxicity Threshold: Above this level, the dose of analgesic induces sedation and respiratory depression.

Pain Relief Threshold: Above this dose threshold, the patient begins to experience pain relief. Below this level, the patient's pain is poorly controlled or uncontrolled.

Figure 6-1. Pattern of pain control when analgesics are administered "as needed" (prn).

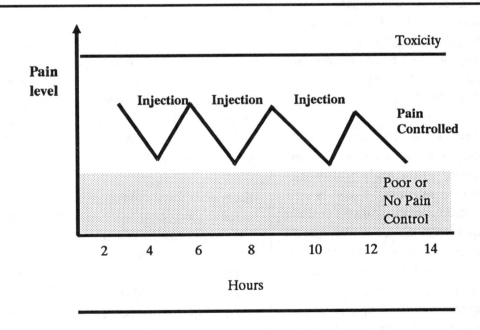

Figure 6-2. Pattern of pain control·when analgesics are administered on a regular schedule to prevent moderate to severe pain.

mation will return along with the pain if the drug is stopped too soon.)

On the other hand, if the NSAID is being taken for its effect against prostaglandins (e.g., for dysmenorrhea) then taking the drug as needed for pain is fine. It is not necessary to maintain a steady blood level of the drug except when the pain is continuing.

Another situation in which it is useful to know the mechanism of analgesia is when advising someone about the selection of over-the-counter analgesic medications for minor discomfort. If the probable source of the pain and the mechanisms of action of the available analgesics are known, it will be clear whether a strong antiinflammatory or a strong anti-prostaglandin effect is needed and whether the drugs should be taken as needed for pain or on a routine basis for several days to reduce inflammation.

Q: Why do orders sometimes call for more than one drug to be given at the same time?

A: Using two drugs instead of one to enhance analgesia without increasing adverse effects is a useful strategy. The drugs, called coanalgesics, are of two main types: (1) those with little or no intrinsic analgesic properties and (2) those that are analgesic but have different mechanisms of action.

The first type includes anxiolytics, antidepressants, and anticonvulsants. Anxiolytics improve the effectiveness of the administered analgesics by reducing a patient's excess tension and anxiety. If used in sufficiently high doses, anxiolytics cause drowsiness and sleep. Nurses should keep in mind, however, that the first antianxiety agent to be used in the acute pain situation is adequate pain relief. Antidepressants are rarely used as coanalgesics in patients with acute pain. Their use is generally for treating chronic pain. Anticonvulsants are also used as coanalgesics in special circumstances to improve pain relief. They are rarely used in cases of acute pain.

For the second type of coanalgesia, most often a nonopioid analgesic is combined with an opioid analgesic. For example, a combination of acetaminophen and codeine is common. The rationale for this combination is that enhanced analgesia is provided without increased side effects such as drowsiness or constipation.

Coanalgesia and a related concept, opioid potentiation, are discussed in more detail in later chapters.

PROBLEM-SOLVING EXERCISES

The following problems are provided so readers can test their understanding of the concepts presented in this chapter. Answering the questions before reading the accompanying discussion is encouraged.

Problem 1

Your patient has been receiving regular doses of oral methadone for the past 4 days to control severe pain caused by cancer. His pain control has been improving steadily, and until today he has had no troublesome side effects. Now he appears lethargic and unsteady on his feet. What problems should be considered in this case?

Discussion. You should check the chart to make certain that the patient has been receiving the proper doses of methadone and that his kidney function is not impaired. However, the most likely explanation is that the patient's blood level of methadone has been increasing steadily during the past 4 days and has reached an excessive level. (Remember, methadone has a long half-life.) The solution is to discuss the situation with the patient's physician, who will probably reduce the daily dose of methadone by increasing the time between doses.

Problem 2

After an intramuscular injection of 75 mg of meperidine, your new postoperative patient had good pain control for approximately 30 min. It is now 2 hr since the last dose, and she is complaining of pain again. Her doctor ordered "meperidine 75–100 mg every 2-4 hr as needed for pain." What will you do?

Discussion. The patient should be given another dose of meperidine as soon as possible to get her pain back under control. Because the 75-mg dose provided only 30 min of good pain relief, the dose should be increased to 100 mg. Subsequent doses should be given every 2–3 hr as long as the patient appears to need that level of analgesia to control her pain. Alternatively, you might consider asking the physician to switch the patient to a longer-acting analgesic, such as morphine, or placing her on a PCA pump so that she can control her own analgesia.

SUMMARY

Uncontrolled pain can undercut efforts to treat a patient's underlying disease. Advances in knowledge about the pharmacology of analgesics mean that adequate relief of patients' pain is possible, and health professionals should be held accountable for providing that relief. Analgesics are categorized into two groups: opioids and nonopioids. Guidelines for the administration of analgesics depend on the specifics of each drug and how these medications control pain. The route of administration, relative potency, time of peak analgesia, and the half-life and mechanism of each drug must be considered. Information on the patient's response to analgesics, the best time to administer the drugs, and use of PCA and coanalgesia are also important. The next chapter provides more material on analgesics.

EXAM QUESTIONS

Chapter 6

Questions 31–38

31. Health professionals most often do not administer available opioid analgesics because they fear which side effect of these drugs?

    a. Drug addiction
    b. Respiratory depression
    c. Urinary retention
    d. Drowsiness

32. How do opioid analgesics reduce pain?

    a. They block the synthesis of prostaglandins.
    b. They bind to opiate receptors in the central nervous system.
    c. They cause the release of endorphins.
    d. They act directly on injured tissues.

33. How do nonopioid analgesics reduce pain?

    a. They block the synthesis of prostaglandins.
    b. They reduce transmission of pain impulses.
    c. They cause the release of endorphins.
    d. They bind to opiate receptors in the central nervous system.

34. What should be the route of administration of an analgesic if the goal is to relieve a patient's pain as quickly as posssible?

    a. Intravenous
    b. Oral
    c. Intramuscular
    d. Subcutaneous

35. What is a major side effect of opioid analgesics?

    a. Decreased alertness
    b. Gastritis
    c. Increased bleeding time
    d. Kidney damage

36. You have just given a patient an intramuscular injection of 10 mg of morphine. How soon, in minutes, would you expect the patient to begin feeling some pain relief?

    a. 5–10
    b. 10–15
    c. 15–30
    d. 30–45

37. What is the duration, in hours, of the analgesic effect of 10 mg of morphine administered intramuscularly?

    a. 1–2
    b. 2–3
    c. 3–5
    d. 4–7

38. How many milligrams of meperidine given intramuscularly is equivalent in analgesic effect to 10 mg of morphine given by the same route?

    a. 25
    b. 50
    c. 75
    d. 100

CHAPTER 7

APPROPRIATE USE OF ANALGESICS FOR VARIOUS LEVELS OF PAIN

CHAPTER OBJECTIVE

After studying this chapter, the reader will be able to discuss the drugs used for moderate to severe pain, the advantages and disadvantages of their use, and their major side effects.

LEARNING OBJECTIVES

After studying this chapter, the reader will be able to

1. Recognize mild to moderate pain and moderate to severe pain on the Visual Analogue Scale.

2. Specify the disadvantages of the different types of aspirin preparations and when their use is contraindicated.

3. Indicate the advantages and disadvantages of the use of acetaminophen over aspirin.

4. Specify major side effects of nonopioid and opioid-containing drugs.

5. Name an opioid-containing combination and an agonist-antagonist drug used for moderate to severe pain.

6. Recognize the correct definitions for tolerance and drug addiction.

INTRODUCTION

Analgesic medications are the most popular method of treating pain in the United States. Therefore, it is important that all health care professionals be thoroughly familiar with the proper use of these drugs. This chapter covers use of analgesics in the treatment of acute pain of various intensities.

MILD TO MODERATE PAIN

What is meant by the term *mild to moderate pain?* How intense is it? Unfortunately, no quantitative definitions are available in the pain literature. For the purposes of this text, mild to moderate pain is defined as pain that has an intensity between 2 and 5 as determined with the Visual Analogue Scale (Figure 7-1). The intensity is 3 most of the time, with occasional fluctuations down to 1 and up to 5. Acute pain means pain that has been a problem for fewer than 6 weeks and is not progressing.

Over-the-Counter Analgesics

During 1988, it was estimated that the American public would spend, that year alone, nearly $2 billion on over-the-counter (OTC) pain relievers. Because of the phenomenal profits to be made in this massive market, drug advertisers work overtime to persuade the consumer that their analgesic products are vastly superior to those offered by competitors. Among the advertising claims made by these manufacturers in the past, the advisory committee of the Food and Drug Administration (FDA) judged that the following were false or misleading:

- Acts five times faster than aspirin
- Arthritis pain formula
- Arthritis strength
- Long-lasting pain relief
- So gentle it can be taken on an empty stomach

The effectiveness of most oral analgesics for the treatment of mild to moderate pain is measured against the effectiveness of 650 mg of aspirin (two adult aspirin tablets). Table 7-1 lists the equianalgesic doses for a variety of analgesics (not all OTC) used for mild to moderate pain.

Most persons, including health care professionals, underestimate the potency of many OTC analgesics. Actually, these drugs can be quite effective in the treatment of pain. Perhaps their potency is discounted because they are so familiar and easily available. Nevertheless, when used properly, they effectively relieve pain that has an intensity of 2–4.

Abuse of Nonopioid Analgesics

In contrast to opioid abuse and addiction, chronic use of nonopioid analgesics has received little or no publicity and attention. Exact numbers on the frequency of abuse of OTC analgesics are not available. Abuse in this respect is defined as regular daily intake of analgesics that results in (1) drug tolerance; that is, increased doses are required to relieve pain and (2) signs and symptoms of withdrawal after the discontinuation of daily medication (Dichgans & Diener, 1988). This type of drug abuse is rarely recognized as a health problem, most likely because these OTC medications are considered so safe. Unfortunately, their abuse can have serious detrimental effects.

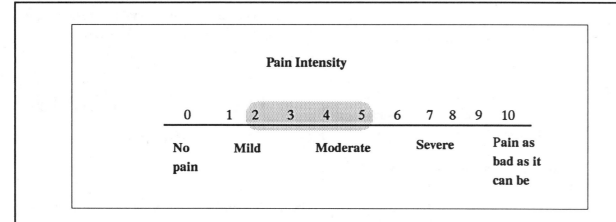

Figure 7-1. Mild to moderate pain on the Visual Analogue Scale.

TABLE 7-1
Equianalgesic Doses of Oral Analgesics Used for Mild to Moderate Pain

Analgesic	Dose (mg)
Nonopioid	
Acetominophen	650
Aspirin	650
Sodium salicylate	1000
Opioid	
Codeine	32
Meperidine (Demerol)	50
Pentazocine (Talwin)	30
Propoxyphene hydrochloride (Darvon)	65
Propoxyphene napsylate (Darvon-N)	100

Physicians experienced in the treatment of chronic pain syndromes such as headache are well aware that the daily intake of antipyretic or antiinflammatory analgesics or combinations containing ergotamine can have adverse effects. Signs and symptoms that suggest abuse of nonopioid analgesics are listed in Table 7-2.

Acetylsalicylic Acid (Aspirin)

Aspirin is still the most commonly used OTC analgesic. It is available plain; buffered; in effervescent tablets or powders; and in combination with other analgesics, antacids, antihistamines, decongestants, and special ingredients that are supposed to enhance its effectiveness.

Despite the many claims of manufacturers, no well-substantiated differences have been found in the effectiveness of different brands of 325-mg tablets of aspirin, even the buffered variety. Great differences in price, however, have been substantiated. The price of Anacin, the most heavily promoted single product in the entire OTC market, is almost six times higher than the price of a generic tablet of aspirin. Anacin does contain more acetylsalicylic acid (ASA) than other brands (400 mg/tablet instead of the usual 325 mg/tablet). It also contains caffeine, the same amount as a quarter of a cup of coffee.

Aspirin is effective in relieving discomfort caused by a wide variety of common disorders: colds, flu, minor arthritis, muscle strains, headaches, and joint pain. In higher doses, it can be effective in relieving pain from more severe arthritis. Aspirin is also used for its reliable antipyretic effects.

Because it is a potent inhibitor of blood clotting, aspirin is now being recommended to many patients who are at increased risk for myocardial infarction. As little as one tablet every other day is thought to be sufficient to maintain this anticlotting effect. A recent study also showed that a small dose of aspirin every other day reduces the number of deaths due to colon cancer. Whether this is due to earlier diagnosis of tumors because aspirin irritates the lesions and causes them to bleed sooner or to some other mechanism is not clear.

Heartburn and other forms of gastric pain and distress occur in 5% of all persons who take aspirin. It is estimated that between 30% and 40% of all cases

---

TABLE 7-2
Signs and Symptoms Suggestive of Abuse of Nonopiod Analgesics

Gastrointestinal Disorders
Gastric ulcers, indigestion, nausea, and vomiting associated with use of analgesics containing aspirin or antiinflammatory medications.

Hematological Disorders
Reduced platelet aggregation as a consequence of use of aspirin or antiinflammatory drugs. May cause chronic loss of blood in urine or stools, causing iron deficiency anemia. Aplastic anemia and agranulocytosis are rare consequences of use of antiinflammatory drugs.

Nephropathy
Due to long-term use of high doses of phenacetin contained in some analgesic combinations.

Dependency
Analgesic preparations that contain caffeine may cause dependeny on the analgesic because of the effects of the accompanying caffeine: increased vigilance, decreased fatigue, and improved performance and mood. Signs and symptoms of caffeine withdrawal are irritability, nervousness, restlessness, and, especially, "caffeine withdrawal headache."

---

of bleeding ulcers that require hospital admission are caused in part by salicylates. Some stomach bleeding occurs in more than half of all persons who take aspirin.

Long-term use of aspirin or products containing aspirin can cause gastritis and microscopic blood loss from the bowel. Some evidence suggests that the use of buffered aspirin minimizes this side effect. Enteric-coated tablets (e.g., A.S.A. Enseals and Ecotrin) are formulated to prevent gastric irritation. However, the tablets do not always dissolve properly and thus provide uneven pain relief. Occasionally, an undissolved tablet is found in the stool. Because the cumulative loss of blood can be sufficient to cause iron deficiency anemia, it is recommended that patients on long-term ASA therapy have their hemoglobin level or hematocrit checked every few months.

Effervescent aspirin solutions. Effervescent aspirin solutions are made by dropping an effervescent aspirin preparation into water. The solution produced by the resulting chemical reaction has not been shown to be more effective than an equivalent dose of aspirin tablets.

Aspirin-containing chewing gum. Aspirin-containing chewing gums (e.g., Aspergum) are not recommended by medical consultants. An FDA advisory panel on internal analgesics has specifically warned against patients' using chewable ASA and ASA-containing gum during the first week after any oral surgery, including tonsillectomy. Aspirin has no proved analgesic effect on mucous membranes, and particles of the medication (i.e., ASA) can cause irritation.

Generic aspirin. Most pharmacies and other retail stores sell house brands of aspirin tablets that are much cheaper than the nationally advertised brands. No evidence indicates that these generic brands are less effective than the more expensive brands. The only problem has been that some of the cheaper tablets may not dissolve as quickly in liquids. Any brand can be tested by dropping one of the tablets in a glass of water and seeing if the tablet dissolves.

Buffered aspirin. Aspirin compounds that include small amounts of antacid are supposed to be less irritating to the stomach because they are less acid. However, use of buffered aspirin has not been shown to actually decrease the prevalence of gastrointestinal upsets. The claim that Bufferin helps prevent the stomach upset often caused by aspirin has not held up to investigation by the Panel on Drugs for Relief of Pain, National Academy of Sciences–National Research Council. The panel concluded that there is little difference in the prevalence or intensity of subjective gastrointestinal side effects after ingestion of Bufferin or plain aspirin. Some studies done by manufacturers have shown that buffered aspirin is absorbed slightly more rapidly than plain aspirin. However, the FDA found no basis for Bufferin's claim that their tablet works twice as fast as aspirin.

Combinations containing aspirin. On the premise that more is better, the aspirin industry has introduced a number of formulations containing a combination of chemicals. The advantages offered by these combinations are often obscure. For example, Excedrin combines aspirin with acetaminophen. As these last two drugs are equianalgesic, it is not clear what advantage Excedrin offers over two tablets of aspirin or two tablets of acetaminophen. Finally, Excedrin adds a small amount of caffeine for good measure (and additional money). Vanquish goes even further toward the shotgun approach, combining aspirin, acetaminophen, caffeine, and small amounts of two antacids.

In response to the tendency for manufacturers to continue adding more ingredients to their pain relievers, the FDA advisory panel on internal analgesics said that, in general, the fewer ingredients in OTC products, the safer the therapy. The American Pharmaceutical Association has also advised against combining several drugs. Its *Handbook of Nonprescription Drugs* advises that combinations containing several analgesic ingredients often imply to consumers that better pain relief will be provided. However, it warns, these claims only confuse the consumer because combinations have not been proved more effective than the sum of their individual ingredients.

Recommendations on administration of aspirin include the following:

* Take the drug with a full glass of water or other liquid.

* Unless instructed by a physician, do not take more than 10 or 15 grains (two or three tablets) at a time, do not take the drug more often than every 4 hr, and do not take more than 10 tablets in 24 hr.

Contraindications. Reye's (pronounced RIZE) syndrome is a rare but frequently fatal disease that affects the central nervous system and liver of persons less than 18 years old. Its development has been linked to use of aspirin in young persons who have chickenpox or influenza. Since 1986, the FDA has required a warning label on aspirin that states that children and teenagers should take aspirin only with the consent of a physician because of the danger of Reye's syndrome.

Another change in aspirin labeling was proposed by the FDA in November 1988. A panel review of bleeding problems caused by medications containing aspirin concluded that women who use aspirin in the last 3 months of their pregnancies have a significant risk of bleeding. Such bleeding, the FDA said, can increase the time a woman spends in labor and may adversely affect bleeding and clotting in both the mother and the newborn. The new aspirin warning label would read as follows: IMPORTANT: Do not take this product during the last 3 months of pregnancy unless directed by a doctor.

Other contraindications and precautions about aspirin are listed in Appendix B.

Acetaminophen

Acetaminophen was developed to take the place of aspirin for those persons for whom aspirin is contraindicated. It is less irritating to the gastric mucosa and does not decrease platelet aggregation, but it does not have aspirin's antiinflammatory effect. Milligram for milligram, aspirin and acetaminophen are equianalgesic.

Overdoses of acetaminophen can be highly toxic to the liver, and prompt treatment is necessary to prevent severe liver damage. Unfortunately, the person usually feels well for as long as 2 days after the overdose. As few as three extra strength Tylenol tablets can be fatal to a child. In November 1988, the FDA proposed stronger labeling on acetaminophen bottles: In case of accidental overdose, contact a physician immediately.

If given in high doses long term, acetaminophen can exhaust the enzyme system in the liver responsible for the drug's breakdown. It can also destroy the liver's ability to break down other toxic substances.

Ibuprofen

Before 1984, ibuprofen could not be purchased without a physician's prescription. At that time, this potent antiinflammatory drug was the fifth most commonly prescribed drug in the United States and was being taken by nearly 7 million persons in this country. Although prescriptions are still required for tablets containing larger amounts of ibuprofen (Motrin and Rufen), tablets containing 200mg of the drug can be bought OTC. Like aspirin, ibuprofen is effective for relief of minor aches and pains associated with minor illnesses and injuries, fever reduction, and relief of specific discomforts such as dysmenorrhea. As already mentioned, it is a potent antiinflammatory. It is not safe for persons who are allergic to aspirin. The contraindications and precautions for use are similar to those for aspirin.

About 10% of persons experience one of the following signs or symptoms when taking ibuprofen: bloating, diarrhea or constipation, dizziness, headache, indigestion, loss of appetite, nausea and/or vomiting, and nervousness. Some say that the OTC doses of ibuprofen offer no advantages over equal amounts of aspirin. The usual OTC dose is one 200-mg tablet every 4–6 hr. Two tablets can be taken at a time, but the likelihood of side effects increases. If more than six tablets a day are being taken for more than a week, the advice of a physician should be sought.

In 1990, pharmaceutical companies began to replace acetaminophen and aspirin with ibuprofen in some of the drug combinations sold for the treatment of colds and sinus problems. This change should provide no special advantages, but it is certainly intended as a method of getting more attention for "new" and "improved" products.

Other Nonsteroidal Antiinflammatory Drugs

As mentioned in chapter 6, NSAIDs provide effective pain relief by acting on the injured or affected tissue. This category of drugs, unless contraindicated, should be used to treat mild to moderate pain. Most NSAIDs increase the risk of bleeding. The risk of gastrointestinal blood loss is also increased slightly. Currently, one NSAID, ketorolac tromethamine (Toradol), has been approved by the FDA for parenteral use. Table 7-3 contains dosing data for commonly used NSAIDs.

MODERATE PAIN

Only the weaker opioids should be used to treat pain of moderate intensity. If these analgesics, taken properly, are not sufficient to control a patient's pain, then the pain is probably more severe than previously supposed or tolerance has developed.

Most of the opioids used for treating moderate pain are actually combinations of coanalgesics: an opioid plus a nonopioid (see Table 7-4). As mentioned in chapter 6, combining analgesics with other medications is an excellent way to increase analgesia without increasing side effects. Unfortunately, some analgesics are combined with chemicals that do not add appreciably to the overall analgesic effect but do add to the number of problems experienced and add considerably to the cost.

MODERATE TO SEVERE PAIN

As is the case with mild to moderate pain, the literature does not provide quantifiable terms for *moderate to severe pain.* For the purposes of this text, moderate to severe pain is defined as pain that has an intensity of 6–10 on the Visual Analogue Scale (Figure 7-2).

Status of Pain Control

Bonica (1987) reviewed the advances made in the control of moderate to severe pain over the previous decade and discussed the extent to which the available information and skills are being applied throughout the world. He found that although tremendous advances had been made, inadequate or improper application of available knowledge and therapies was the most important reason for current deficiencies.

The identified causes responsible for improper application of available knowledge about potent analgesics included the following:

- Lack of organized teaching of medical students, physicians, nurses, and other health professionals about the clinical management of patients with acute and chronic pain

- Inadequate sources of other information such as books and journals available for the education of students and practitioners

The available evidence suggests that this deficiency in medical education and training has been due to a lack of, or insufficient interest and concern by, medical educators. Some schools of nursing have improved their education in pain management, but a brief review of several critical care textbooks and other continuing education resources for nurses

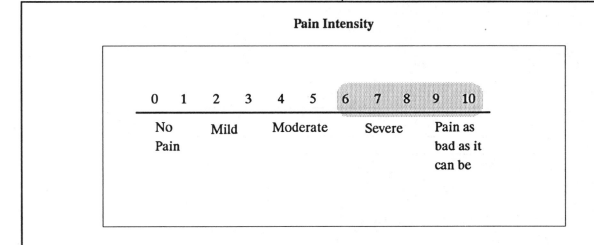

Figure 7-2. Moderate to severe pain on the Visual Analogue Scale.

Table 7-3
Dosing Data for NSAIDs

Drug	Usual adult dose	Usual pediatric dose[1]	Comments
Oral NSAIDs			
Acetaminophen	650–975 mg q 4 hr	10–15 mg/kg q 4 hr	Acetaminophen lacks the peripheral anti-inflammatory activity of other NSAIDs
Aspirin	650–975 mg q 4 hr	10–15 mg/kg q 4 hr[2]	The standard against which other NSAIDs are compared. Inhibits platelet aggregation; may cause postoperative bleeding
Choline magnesium trisalicylate (Trilisate)	1000–1500 mg bid	25 mg/kg bid	May have minimal antiplatelet activity; also available as oral liquid
Diflunisal (Dolobid)	1000 mg initial dose followed by 500 mg q 12 hr		
Etodolac (Lodine)	200–400 mg q 6–8 hr		
Fenoprofen calcium (Nalfon)	200 mg q 4–6 hr		
Ibuprofen (Motrin, others)	400 mg q 4–6 hr	10 mg/kg q 6–8 hr	Available as several brand names and as generic; also available as oral suspension
Ketoprofen (Orudis)	25–75 mg q 6–8 hr		
Magnesium salicylate	650 mg q 4 hr		Many brands and generic forms available

Drug	Usual adult dose	Usual pediatric dose[1]	Comments
Oral NSAIDs			
Meclofenamate sodium (Meclomen)	50 mg q 4–6 hr		
Mefenamic acid (Ponstel)	250 mg q 6 hr		
Naproxen (Naprosyn)	500 mg initial dose followed by 250 mg q 6–8 hr	5 mg/kg q 12 hr	Also available as oral liquid
Naproxen sodium (Anaprox)	550 mg initial dose followed by 275 mg q 6–8 hr		
Salsalate (Disalcid, others)	500 mg q 4 hr		May have minimal antiplatelet activity
Sodium salicylate	325–650 mg q 3–4 hr		Available in generic form from several distributors

Drug	Usual adult dose	Usual pediatric dose[1]	Comments
Parenteral NSAID			
Ketorolac	30 or 60 mg IM initial dose followed by 15 or 30 mg q 6 hr Oral dose following IM dosage: 10 mg q 6–8 hr		Intramuscular dose not to exceed 5 days

Note: Only the above NSAIDs have FDA approval for use as simple analgesics, but clinical experience has been gained with other drugs as well.

[1] Drug recommendations are limited to NSAIDs where pediatric dosing experience is available.

[2] Contraindicated in presence of fever or other evidence of viral illness.

TABLE 7-4
Combination Analgesics for Moderate Pain

Agent	Dose Equivalent to 650 mg ASA (mg)
Codeine	32

Ascodeen-30
[codeine 30 mg + acetylsalicylic acid (ASA) 325 mg]

Ascriptin with codeine #2*
[codeine 16 mg + ASA 325 mg + Maalox 150 mg]

Acriptin with codeine #3
[codeine 32 mg + ASA 325 mg + Maalox 150 mg]

Empirin compound with codeine #1**
[codeine 7.5 mg + ASA 225 mg + phenacetin 162 mg +caffeine 32 mg]

Empirin compound with codeine #2
[codeine 15 mg + ASA 225 mg + phenacetin 162 mg + caffeine 32 mg]

Empirin compound with codeine #3

Phenaphen with codeine #3
[codeine 30 mg + ASA 225 mg + phenacetin 162 mg + caffeine 32 mg]

Empirin compound with codeine #4
[codeine 60 mg + ASA 225 mg + phenacetin 162 mg + caffeine 32 mg]

Empracet #3
[codeine 30 mg + acetaminophen 300 mg]

Empracet #4
[codeine 60 mg + acetaminophen 300 mg]

Phenaphen with codeine #2*
[codeine 15 mg + acetaminophen 325 mg]

Phenaphen with codeine #3
[codeine 30 mg + acetaminophen 325 mg]

Phenaphen with codeine #4
[codeine 60 mg + acetaminophen 325 mg]

Tylenol with codeine #1**
[codeine 7.5 mg + acetaminophen 300 mg]

Tylenol with codeine #2
[codeine 15 mg + acetaminophen 300 mg]

TABLE 7-4 (continued)
Combination Analgesics for Moderate Pain

Agent	Dose Equivalent to 650 mg ASA (mg)
Codeine	32
Tylenol with codeine #3 [codeine 30 mg + acetaminophen 300 mg]	
Tylenol with codeine #4 [codeine 60 mg + acetaminophen 300 mg]	
Hydrocodone (Vicodin, Dicodid) [hydrocodone + acetaminophen]	Unknown
Meperidine (Demerol)	
Demerol-APAP [meperidine 50 mg + acetaminophen 300 mg]	
Mepergan Fortis capsules** [meperidine 50 mg + promethazine 25 mg]	
Oxycodone	
Percodan [oxycodone hydrochloride 4.5 mg + oxycodone terephthalate 0.38 mg + ASA 325 mg + phenacetin 160 mg + caffeine 32 mg]	15
Percocet-5 [oxycodone hydrochloride 5 mg + acetaminophen 325 mg]	
Percodan-Demi [oxycodone hydrochloride 2.25 mg+ oxycodone 0.19 mg + ASA 224 mg + phenacetin 160 mg + caffeine 32 mg]	
Pentazocine (Talwin) Talwin Compound [pentazocine 12.5 mg + ASA 325 mg]	30

TABLE 7-4 (continued)
Combination Analgesics for Moderate Pain

Agent	Dose Equivalent to 650 mg ASA (mg)
Propoxyphene (Darvon)	65
Darvon Compound [propoxyphene 32 mg + ASA 227 mg + phenacetin 65 mg + caffeine 32 mg]	
Darvon Compound 65 [propoxyphene 65 mg + ASA 227 mg + phenacetin 65 mg + caffeine 32 mg]	
Darvon with ASA [propoxyphene 65 mg + ASA 325 mg]	
Propoxyphene napsylate (Darvon-N)	100
Darvon-N with ASA [propoxyphene napsylate 100 mg + ASA 325 mg]	
Darvocet-N-50 [propoxyphene napsylate 50 mg + acetaminophen 325 mg]	
Darvocet-N-100 [propoxyphene napsylate 100 mg + acetaminophen 650 mg]	

*Equal to 650 mg of aspirin (2 tablets).

**Provides LESS analgesia than 650 mg of aspirin.

showed that virtually no serious attention is given to this subject.

Nurses in clinical practice also have few clinically relevant educational materials on pain management. Most professionals keep up to date through discussions with their colleagues and by reading professional magazines. Such approaches, however, do not adequately meet the clinical nurse's need for a comprehensive course on pain management.

Guidelines for Analgesic Control

Patients with moderate to severe pain usually require potent analgesics as part of their pain management regimen. These drugs are mostly controlled substances and are classified as opioids. Dosing data for opioid analgesics are summarized in Table 7-5.

Variability of Absorption

The choice of analgesic drug for treating severe acute pain depends, in part, on the possible routes of administration. For example, if a patient is unable to take drugs orally, then a drug that can be given by parenteral routes will be chosen.

Some pharmacokinetic studies of traditional opioids have shown unsuspected variations in drug absorption and excretion. For example, one study of intra-

Table 7-5
Dosing Data for Opioid Analgesics

Drug	Approximate equianalgesic oral dose	Approximate equianalgesic parenteral dose	Recommended starting dose (adults more than 50 kg body weight) oral	parenteral	Recommended starting dose (children and adults less than 50 kg body weight)[1] oral	parenteral
Opioid Agonist						
Morphine[2]	30 mg q 3–4 hr (around-the-clock dosing)	10 mg q 3–4 hr	30 mg q 3–4 hr	10 mg q 3–4 hr	0.3 mg/kg q 3–4 hr	0.1 mg/kg q 3–4 hr
	60 mg q 3–4 hr (single dose or intermittent dosing)					
Codeine[3]	130 mg q 3–4 hr	75 mg q 3–4 hr	60 mg q 3–4 hr	60 mg q 2 hr (intramuscular/subcutaneous)	1 mg/kg q 3–4 hr[4]	Not recommended
Hydromophone[2] (Dilaudid)	7.5 mg q 3–4 hr	1.5 mg q 3–4 hr	6 mg q 3–4 hr	1.5 mg q 3–4 hr	0.06 mg/kg q 3–4 hr	0.015 mg/kg q 3–4 hr
Hydrocodone (in Lorcet, Lortab, Vicodin, others)	30 mg q 3–4 hr	Not available	10 mg q 3–4 hr	Not available	0.2 mg/kg q 3–4 hr[4]	Not available
Levorphanol (Levo-Dromoran)	4 mg q 6–8 hr	2 mg q 6–8 hr	4 mg q 6–8 hr	2 mg q 6–8 hr	0.04 mg/kg q 6–8 hr	0.02 mg/kg q 6–8 hr
Meperidine (Demerol)	300 mg q 2–3 hr	100 mg q 3 hr	Not recommended	100 mg q 3 hr	Not recommended	0.75 mg/kg q 2–3 hr
Methadone (Dolophine, others)	20 mg q 6–8 hr	10 mg q 6–8 hr	20 mg q 6–8 hr	10 mg q 6–8 hr	0.2 mg/kg q 6–8 hr	0.1 mg/kg q 6–8 hr
Oxycodone (Roxicodone, also in Percocet, Percodan, Tylox, others)	30 mg q 3–4 hr	Not available	10 mg q 3–4 hr	Not available	0.2 mg/kg q 3–4 hr[4]	Not available
Oxymorphone[2] (Numorphan)	Not available	1 mg q 3–4 hr	Not available	1 mg q 3-4 hr	Not recommended	Not recommended
Opioid Agonist-Antagonist and Partial Agonist						
Buprenorphine (Buprenex)	Not available	0.3–0.4 mg q 6–8 hr	Not available	0.4 mg q 6–8 hr	Not available	0.004 mg/kg q 6–8 hr
Butorphanol (Stadol)	Not available	2 mg q 3–4 hr	Not available	2 mg q 3–4 hr	Not available	Not recommended
Nalbuphine (Nubain)	Not available	10 mg q 3–4 hr	Not available	10 mg q 3–4 hr	Not available	0.1 mg/kg q 3–4 hr
Pentazocine (Talwin, others)	150 mg q 3–4 hr	60 mg q 3–4 hr	50 mg q 4–6 hr	Not recommended	Not recommended	Not recommended

Note: Published tables vary in the suggested doses that are equianalgesic to morphine. Clinical response is the criterion that must be applied for each patient; titration to clinical response is necessary. Because there is not complete cross tolerance among these drugs, it is usually necessary to use a lower than equianalgesic dose when changing drugs and to retitrate to response.

Caution: Recommended doses do not apply to patients with renal or hepatic insufficiency or other conditions affecting drug metabolism and kinetics.

[1] **Caution:** Doses listed for patients with body weight less than 50 kg cannot be used as initial starting doses in babies less than 6 months of age. Consult the *Clinical Practice Guideline for Acute Pain Management: Operative or Medical Procedures and Trauma* section on management of pain in neonates for recommendations.

[2] For morphine, hydromorphone, and oxymorphone, rectal administration is an alternate route for patients unable to take oral medications, but equianalgesic doses may differ from oral and parenteral doses because of pharmacokinetic differences.

[3] **Caution:** Codeine doses above 65 mg often are not appropriate due to diminishing incremental analgesia with increasing doses but continually increasing constipation and other side effects.

[4] **Caution:** Doses of aspirin and acetaminophen in combination opioid/NSAID preparations must also be adjusted to the patient's body weight.

Source: U.S. Department of Health and Human Services/Public Health Service.

muscular injection of 100 mg of meperidine every 4 hr for postoperative pain showed the following:

- The peak blood concentration of meperidine varied fivefold between patients.

- Within the same patient, the peak concentration varied twofold.

- Pain control was poor during the first 4-hr dosing interval. Good analgesia was not achieved until the third or fourth dose of meperidine was administered.

- Even after good pain relief was finally achieved, the onset of relief was approximately 45 min, and duration was only 75–90 min. The pain then increased steadily to severe levels by the fourth hour after administration.

These findings explain many of the confusing responses seen in the past in patients given meperidine for postoperative pain or before painful procedures.

New Drugs

The past decade has also seen the development of new opioid analgesics, both of the agonist and of the agonist-antagonist types. The newer mixed agonist-antagonist drugs differ significantly from morphine. They resemble morphine in analgesic properties, but resemble nalorphine (Narcan) (antagonists) in their blocking of opioid effects. Therefore, they should never be given to patients being treated with agonists such as morphine. The available evidence indicates that the degree of respiratory depression caused by agonist-antagonist drugs is not dose related. That is, larger doses of these agents do not cause increasing respiratory depression.

Butorphanol (Stadol). The effectiveness of butorphanol, an agonist-antagonist, in the treatment of postoperative pain is comparable to that obtained with morphine, meperidine (Demerol), or pentazocine (Talwin). The most frequently reported adverse reactions are sedation, nausea, and sweating. Other reactions with a prevalence of more than 1% include headache, vertigo, feeling of floating, dizziness, lethargy, confusion, and light-headedness.

Nalbuphine (Nubain). Another agonist-antagonist that provides effective pain control in moderate to severe pain is nalbuphine. The onset of action is 2–3 min after intravenous administration and within 15 min after intramuscular or subcutaneous administration. The effects last 3–6 hr. The major adverse side effect is sedation (one third of patients). Other side effects include a sweaty, clammy feeling; nausea and vomiting; dizziness and vertigo; dryness of the mouth; and headache.

Buprenorphine (Buprenex). Buprenorphine, a partial agonist, is not available in oral form. In the United States, it is available only in its parenteral form; in Europe, it is available in both sublingual and parenteral forms. This drug is most useful as a starting analgesic medication, before patients have been given analgesic agonists. When used in patients receiving opioid agonists, its analgesic efficacy is diminished. The respiratory depressant effects of buprenorphine are not readily reversed by naloxone. Instead, drugs that stimulate the central nervous system must be used.

COMBINING ANALGESICS

Pain medications can be combined in many different ways to increase analgesia with minimum side effects. For example, if a patient has mild to moderate pain most of the time, a nonopioid such as aspirin or acetaminophen can be used on a regular basis, and an opioid can be added when a flare-up of pain occurs. Even if the pain progresses, requiring an opioid analgesic on a regular basis, the nonopioid analgesic can be continued. Combinations of nonopioids with opioids can provide additive analgesia, may reduce side effects, and can reduce the rate at which the dosage of the opioid analgesic must be increased.

Combinations of an opioid plus an antihistamine, specifically hydroxyzine, or an opioid plus an amphetamine, such as Dexedrine, also provide additional analgesia without an increase in the opioid dose being used.

SIDE EFFECTS OF OPIOID ANALGESICS

Many side effects are associated with the use of opioid analgesics. Depending on the situation, these can be categorized as desirable or undesirable. Adverse effects are those that markedly limit use of the drugs. The mechanisms underlying these side effects are not well understood. Influencing factors include age, extent of disease, previous exposure to opioids, and route of administration.

The most common side effects are sedation, nausea and vomiting, constipation, and respiratory depression. In addition, many other side effects, including confusion, hallucinations, nightmares, urinary retention, multifocal myoclonus, dizziness, and dysphoria, may occur with long-term use of opioids.

Respiratory Depression

Respiratory depression is potentially the most serious adverse effect of morphine and morphinelike agonist opioids. It is also the side effect most feared by health care professionals. Respiratory depression usually occurs in patients who have not used opioids before and is accompanied by other signs of depression of the central nervous system, including sedation and mental clouding. Tolerance to this effect develops rapidly with repeated drug administration.

The respiratory depression caused by mixed agonist-antagonists (e.g., pentazocine, nalbuphine, and butorphanol) and partial agonists (e.g., buprenorphine) appears to differ from the depression caused by morphinelike drugs. For example, although therapeutic doses of pentazocine produce respiratory depression equivalent to that caused by morphine, increasing the dose of pentazocine does not ordinarily produce a proportional increase in respiratory depression. It is not clear if this is a clinically useful advantage.

Constipation

Constipation is such a frequent side effect of the use of opioid analgesics that it can be considered almost invariable. These drugs act at multiple sites in the gastrointestinal tract and spinal cord to produce a decrease in intestinal secretions and peristalsis. Dry stools and constipation are the result. Unfortunately, this is one side effect of opioids to which tolerance develops only slowly.

Steps to prevent constipation should be taken at the time opioid therapy begins. Laxatives and stool softeners are usually required. Their doses usually must be increased as the doses of opiates are increased.

Nausea and Vomiting

The extent of nausea and vomiting caused by an opioid analgesic varies from drug to drug and from patient to patient. Tolerance to these two side effects can occur with repeated administration, usually within 24–48 hr. The prevalence of nausea and vomiting is markedly increased in ambulatory patients; the drugs likely alter vestibular sensitivity.

Several approaches are used to control these side effects. Giving an antiemetic with the opioid can be helpful. Switching the patient to another analgesic may also reduce the gastrointestinal distress. Sometimes changing the route of administration is useful.

Urinary Retention

Because the opioid analgesics increase smooth muscle tone, they can cause bladder spasm and an increase in sphincter tone, leading to urinary retention. This is most common in elderly patients. Catheterization may be required.

Development of Addiction

Addiction cannot be discussed without considering two other conditions that occur along with it: *tolerance* and *physical dependence.*

Drug tolerance develops when a given dose of an opioid analgesic produces less analgesia. That is, a larger dose is required to maintain the same level of pain control. Tolerance appears to develop in all patients who use opioids for long periods. The length of time it takes for tolerance to develop varies tremendously from patient to patient. The important fact to remember is that the development of tolerance does not mean that the patient is physically dependent or addicted to the opioid.

The term physical dependence is used to describe the phenomenon of withdrawal that occurs when an opioid is abruptly discontinued or an opioid antagonist is administered. Physical dependence is a biochemical state caused by the long-term administration of narcotics. Persons who are physically dependent have increased anxiety, nervousness, irritability, and alternating chills and hot flushes. A prominent withdrawal sign is "wetness," which includes salivation, lacrimation, rhinorrhea, and diaphoresis as well as gooseflesh. At the peak intensity of withdrawal, patients may have nausea and vomiting, abdominal cramps, insomnia, and, rarely, multifocal myoclonus.

The term addiction cannot be used interchangeably with physical dependence. It is possible to be physically dependent on an opioid-type analgesic without being addicted. Addiction can best be described as a psychological dependence: a pattern of drug use characterized by a continued craving for the drug that is manifested as compulsive drug-seeking behavior leading to an overwhelming involvement with the use and procurement of the drug.

Fear of addiction is the major concern that limits the appropriate use of opioids for patients in pain. Vigilant regulation by the government has further discouraged physicians from prescribing potent opioids. Joranson, a pain expert at the University of Wisconsin Medical School, has found that states that require physicians to use special triplicate prescription pads when prescribing potent opioid analgesics have experienced a 50% drop in the use of these pain medications. In California, which requires these special prescriptions forms, only one in five physicians has applied for the forms. This means that the vast majority of California's physicians cannot prescribe strong analgesics (Roark, 1991).

Some patients are reluctant to take even small doses of opioids for fear of becoming addicted. Recent surveys of hospitalized medical patients and a study of cancer patients on long-term treatment with opioid analgesics suggest that medical use of opioids rarely, if ever, leads to drug abuse or addiction (Foley & Inturrisi, 1990).

Patients with severe pain who become tolerant to and dependent on opioids can be withdrawn from the drugs without excessive distress. The process is to reduce the drug intake slowly. Pain experts, Foley and Inturrisi (1990), recommend the following method for withdrawing patients from high doses of opioids:

> Experience indicates that the usual daily dose required to prevent withdrawal is equal to one fourth of the previous daily dose. This dose, called the detoxification dose, for want of a better term, is given in four divided doses. The initial detoxification dose is given for 2 days and then decreased by one half (administered in four divided doses) for 2 days until a total daily dose of 10 to 15 mg/day is reached. After 2 days on this dose, the opioid can be discontinued. Thus, a patient who had been receiving 240 mg of morphine per day for pain would require an initial detoxification dose of 60 mg given as 15 mg every 6 hours.

Oversedation or Overdose

Perhaps the fear of overdosing patients is even greater than the fear of addicting them. The concern is that respiratory depression will lead to complications such as atelectasis and pneumonia. The ultimate worry is that respiration will cease altogether. In fact, respiratory depression is relatively uncommon, particularly in patients with acute pain. The flight-or-fight response triggered by severe pain is a powerful stimulant to respiration.

Some degree of sedation is an invariable side effect of opioid analgesics. Nurses tend to think that patients who are sleeping deeply for long intervals are oversedated. However, in many instances, the patient is not overmedicated. Instead, he or she is finally getting sufficient sleep. Nurses also sometimes mistakenly think that a patient who is difficult to awaken during the night is oversedated and often delay the patient's next dose of analgesic. Difficulty in awakening a patient is not necessarily a sign of opioid overdose. Patients vary greatly in how easily they can be awakened. Even the same patient can vary from night to night and hour to hour, depending on the level of sleep. If the patient is breathing regularly, even though it may be only six to eight times per minute, the nurse should not be overly concerned about respiratory depression.

Occasionally, patients with an unusually low threshold to the sedative effects of opioids may show signs and symptoms of overdosage. In other instances, an overdose may occur accidentally because the dose used to control overwhelming pain is increased too rapidly or because opioids with long half-lives slowly accumulate. Whatever the cause, the appropriate treatment is the administration of intravenous naloxone (Narcan), usually 0.4 mg in 10 ml of saline. The patient may awaken in a state of total pain and fear, because the naloxone blocks the effects of both exogenous and endogenous opiates.

SUMMARY

When used properly, OTC nonopioid analgesics can be effective and safe for control of mild to moderate pain. Patients should be encouraged to use these drugs before resorting to more powerful prescription analgesics. Prescription-strength NSAIDs are also available to treat mild to moderate pain. Although they have a fairly large margin of safety, these drugs still should be viewed as potentially dangerous and taken with care.

Opioid analgesics and combinations containing opioids are effective for treatment of moderate and moderate to severe pain. Opioids can be combined with nonopioids to increase pain relief without increasing side effects. Respiratory depression and oversedation, two of the most serious side effects associated with the use of opioids, are not as common as most health professionals fear. Patients can become tolerant to and physically dependent on opioids without becoming addicted. Medical use of opioids rarely leads to addiction.

EXAM QUESTIONS

Chapter 7

Questions 39–53

39. Pain with a rating of 4 on the Visual Analogue Scale of pain intensity would be considered what type of pain?

    a. Mild to severe
    b. Mild to moderate
    c. No pain to mild
    d. Moderate to severe

40. What is a major side effect of aspirin-containing nonopioid analgesics?

    a. Drowsiness
    b. Gastritis
    c. Urinary retention
    d. Respiratory depression

41. What is a major advantage of the use of acetaminophen over aspirin?

    a. Increased and more even absorption
    b. Decreased gastric irritation
    c. Increased antiinflammatory effects
    d. Decreased damage to the liver

42. What effect does acetaminophen lack that aspirin has?

    a. Analgesic
    b. Antipyretic
    c. Antiinfective
    d. Antiinflammatory

43. What is a disadvantage of using Aspergum over other aspirin preparations?

    a. Increased oral irritation
    b. Decreased effectiveness
    c. Decreased dosage
    d. Increased stomach irritation

44. What is a disadvantage of using enteric-coated aspirin preparations over nonenteric-coated preparations?

    a. Pain relief is decreased because of decreased potency.
    b. The tablets do not dissolve until they reach the lower bowel.
    c. No real decrease in gastric upset has been found.
    d. Pain relief is uneven because the tablets do not always dissolve properly.

45. Use of aspirin preparations has been linked to the development of what disease?

    a. Meniere's syndrome
    b. Legionnaires' disease
    c. Gilchrist's disease
    d. Reye's syndrome

46. During what stage of pregnancy are all aspirin preparations contraindicated?

    a. Second trimester
    b. First month
    c. Fourth and fifth months
    d. Third trimester

47. What is one of the major side effects caused by large doses of acetaminophen?

    a. Prolonged bleeding
    b. Gastric irritation
    c. Decreased production of erythrocytes
    d. Liver damage

48. Which of the following is an opioid-containing combination used for moderate to severe pain?

    a. Rufen
    b. Enseals
    c. Motrin
    d. Empracet

49. What is defined as the body adapting to an opioid analgesic so that over time the drug becomes less and less effective in relieving pain?

    a. Addiction
    b. Physical dependence
    c. Psychological dependence
    d. Tolerance

50. Which of the following is an agonist-antagonist drug used for moderate to severe pain?

    a. Empracet
    b. Talwin
    c. Oxycodone
    d. Stadol

51. What is one of the major side effects caused by opioid-containing analgesics?

    a. Hallucinations
    b. Constipation
    c. Vertigo
    d. Headache

52. How is moderate to severe pain rated on the Visual Analogue Scale?

    a. 1–3
    b. 2–5
    c. 4–7
    d. 6–10

53. What is defined as overwhelming involvement with obtaining and using a drug and a strong tendency to return to this behavior after being withdrawn from the drug?

    a. Physical dependence
    b. Addiction
    c. Psychological tolerance
    d. Tolerance

CHAPTER 8

MANAGEMENT OF ACUTE PAIN

CHAPTER OBJECTIVE

After studying this chapter, the reader will be able to state the prevalence of postoperative pain, descriptions used for pain, and the results of inadequate and adequate pain treatment.

LEARNING OBJECTIVES

After studying this chapter, the reader will be able to

1. Specify a biochemical substance known to increase the responsiveness of peripheral pain receptors after injury.

2. Specify the type of surgery most likely to cause severe to moderate postoperative pain and the most common complication associated with undertreatment of this pain.

3. Indicate how many postoperative patients in a group of 10 can be expected to complain of pain and how many will report pain relief with 10 mg of morphine.

4. Recognize the words that a patient might use to describe somatic and incisional pain.

5. Indicate the physiological results of uncontrolled postoperative pain.

6. Specify the percentage of ordered analgesics nurses tend to administer to patients.

7. Indicate an advantage for the use of patient-controlled analgesia and intraspinal opioids.

INTRODUCTION

Acute pain consists of a constellation of unpleasant physical and emotional sensations and associated autonomic reflex responses and psychological and behavioral reactions (Bonica, 1987). Nearly always, this type of pain and its associated responses are triggered by tissue-damaging injury or disease. Although psychological factors have a profound influence on the perception of acute pain, psychopathologic conditions are rarely the primary cause (Bonica, 1988). This is a major difference between acute and chronic pain. The pathophysiology of acute pain is relatively well understood, and its diagnosis is usually straightforward, unlike in chronic pain situations. With effective therapy or because of the self-limiting nature of the disease or the healing of injury, acute pain and its associated responses disappear within days or weeks.

TISSUE INJURY

Tissue destruction, whether from crush injury, fracture, surgery, or a disease, causes certain predictable physiological responses. The local and systemic changes caused by cell damage and the circulatory, ventilatory, and metabolic changes produced by segmental and suprasegmental reflexes may lead to dysfunction of vital organs and produce numerous complications (See chapter 5, Figure 5-1, Pain cycle in unrelieved acute pain). This chapter reviews the physiology of pain already discussed in chapter 3 and presents more detailed information on acute pain.

Peripheral Pain Receptors

Pain is usually initiated by stimulation of peripheral pain receptors (nociceptors) or afferent nerve fibers. In cutaneous nerves, close to half of the sensory fibers originate from peripheral pain receptors. As described in chapter 3, these are A delta and C fibers. Pain messages are transmitted rapidly by the thin myelinated A delta fibers and more slowly by the thick unmyelinated C fibers. Sensations carried by A delta fibers are described as sharp and well localized. Sensations carried by C fibers, on the other hand, are dull, burning, and poorly localized.

Factors That Increase the Responsiveness of Pain Receptors

A number of factors increase the responsiveness of peripheral pain receptors after injury (i.e., lower the threshold for firing). When tissue is injured, biochemical substances released into the surrounding area sensitize the peripheral receptors so that even minor stimuli trigger the transduction and subsequent transmission of pain sensations. These substances include the following:

- Potassium (K^+): produces pain in the damaged tissues for various lengths of time.

- Acetylcholine (ACh): lowers the threshold for other pain-producing substances.

- Histamine: produces deep pain when applied to deep layers of tissue.

- Serotonins: are released during the process of blood coagulation.

- Plasma kinins: develop in blood plasma at the site of injury.

These substances also increase the sensations of pain indirectly by increasing vasoconstriction, which decreases the microcirculatory blood supply.

Other pain-inducing substances produced by the body in response to tissue injury are prostaglandins. Prostaglandins are derived from the essential fatty acid, arachidonic acid, which appears to be generated by all tissues. These compounds contribute significantly to the pain and swelling associated with inflammation. In addition to lowering the threshold of nerve endings to noxious mechanical and chemical stimuli (thus promoting tenderness), they cause vasodilatation, leading to redness, increased swelling, and further tissue damage.

Segmental and Suprasegmental Spinal Reflexes

Segmental and suprasegmental spinal reflexes are the result of pain-induced stimulation of regions within the spinal cord and hypothalamus. These reflexes can, and often do, intensify the perception of pain. In addition, hyperactivity of the sympathetic nervous system and the consequent liberation of norepinephrine into the circulation cause many of the signs and symptoms characteristic of acute pain:

- Increased skeletal muscle tension: decreases chest compliance and initiates feedback, causing more pain messages to be sent from muscles.

- Hyperventilation.

- Increase in heart rate and stroke volume: results in increased myocardial oxygen consumption and work load.

- Decreased gastrointestinal tone: may produce ileus.

- Increased blood pressure.

- Vasoconstriction.

- Decreased urinary output.

The degree and duration of endocrine and metabolic changes are related to the degree and duration of tissue damage. Many biochemical changes last for days and lead to a catabolic state and negative nitrogen balance.

Cortical Responses

Cortical responses include not only the sensation of pain but also the triggering of emotions such as anxiety, apprehension, and fear. These intense emotions can greatly increase the amount of cortisol and catecholamine released into the systemic circulation. Anxiety can even cause cortically mediated increases in blood viscosity, clotting time, fibrinolysis, and platelet aggregation.

POSTOPERATIVE PAIN

Prevalence

The prevalence of moderate to severe pain after surgery is not precisely known, and the occurrence of such pain in a given patient is not predictable. Some information is available, however, about the types of operations most likely to cause moderate to severe pain (Table 8-1). For example, incisions involving the thoracic, upper abdominal, and abdominal cavities are said to produce the most intense and prolonged pain postoperatively. Next most painful, in order, are anorectal surgery and operations involving the back (Bonica, 1982).

In general, several studies showed the following:

- Nearly 4 in 10 (40%) of all postoperative patients never complain of pain.

- One in 5 patients (20%) reports relief of pain with doses of morphine of 10 mg or less.

- Slightly more than 1 in 10 patients (11%) require more than 10-mg doses of morphine for relief of pain.

- One in 5 patients (20%) experiences pain relief with placebos.

- Slightly fewer than 1 in 10 patients never receive adequate pain relief.

Importance of Adequate Postoperative Pain Control

As discussed earlier, further tissue damage occurs if acute pain is allowed to persist. Postoperative pain should be controlled not only because it results in unnecessary suffering but also because it sets up a pain feedback loop, increasing the likelihood that complications will develop.

In addition to the endogenous pain-producing substances released and produced as a result of tissue injury, mechanical mechanisms increase the amount of postoperative pain:

- Distension
- Spasm
- Obstruction
- Edema

TABLE 8-1
Intensity and Duration of Postoperative Pain After Various Operations

Site or Type of Operation	Steady Wound Pain (%)			Mean Duration of Moderate to Severe Pain in Days (Range)
	Minimal	Moderate	Severe	
Thoracotomy	5–15	25–35	60–70	4 (2–7)
Gastrectomy	5–20	20–30	50–75	3 (2–6)
Cholecystectomy	10–20	25–35	45–65	2 (1–5)
Hysterectomy	15–25	30–40	35–55	2 (1–4)
Colectomy, appendectomy	15–25	30–40	20–30	1 (0.5–3)
Nephrectomy, pyelolithotomy	5–15	10–15	70–85	5 (3–7)
Laminectomy	5–10	15–20	70–80	4 (2–7)
Hip(replacement)	5–10	20–30	60–70	3 (2–6)
Shoulder/elbow reconstruction	15–20	25–35	45–60	3 (2–6)
Major hand or foot	10–15	15–20	65–70	3 (2–6)
Open reduction, graft/amputation	10–15	20–30	55–70	2 (1–4)
Closed reduction	30–35	40–50	15–30	1 (0.5–3)
Vascular	30–40	35–40	20–35	1.5 (1–3)
Bladder and prostate	10–15	15–20	65–75	1 (0.5–4)
Anorectal	15–20	25–30	50–60	2 (1–5)
Vaginal	15–55	35–40	15–20	1 (0.5–3)
Scrotal	30–40	35–45	15–35	1 (0.5–3)
Maxillofacial	20–30	25–35	35–55	2 (1–6)
Ventral hernia	30–40	35–45	15–25	1.5 (1–3)
Minor mastectomy	45–50	40–45	5–15	0.5 (0–1)

Source: Bonica, 1982.

- Traction
- Contraction
- Stretching
- Tearing
- Inflammation
- Infection
- Pressure (intraabdominal or compressive)

During surgery, the cortical responses are impaired or completely eliminated by the anesthetic. The segmental and suprasegmental spinal reflexes, although impaired to some degree, can still be triggered by noxious stimuli. However, as the effects of anesthesia fade, the injured tissues trigger pain responses, primarily by releasing pain-inducing substances into the surrounding tissues.

Types of Postoperative Pain

Most patients experience three types of postoperative pain: (1) incisional or cutaneous, (2) somatic, and (3) visceral.

Incisional pain. Every patient who undergoes a major operation is expected to experience some degree of incisional pain. This pain is due to trauma to skin and mucous membranes during surgery and is produced by both mechanical and chemical mechanisms. Most commonly, patients describe this type of pain as sharp, cutting, stabbing, tearing, burning, or full of pressure. Incisional pain is generally transmitted by the thin A delta fibers.

The intensity of incisional pain is affected by the factors listed in Table 8-2. Nurses should consider these factors when planning a patient's postoperative care.

Somatic pain. Somatic pain arises from injured muscles, tendons, ligaments, peritoneum, bone, joints, and arteries (McQuay, Carroll, & Moore, 1988). It is produced by both chemical and mechanical mechanisms and is characterized by a dull, aching discomfort that is difficult to localize, particularly when it involves the thoracic or abdominal regions. The most significant aspect of somatic pain is its tendency to spread and envelop wide areas of the body. Somatic pain is generally carried by the thick C fibers.

Visceral pain. Visceral pain is associated with visceral organs, the peritoneum, or the pleura. Like somatic pain, it is characterized as dull and aching, but it has different manifestations, depending on the intensity and duration of the noxious stimulus. For example, visceral pain of abdominal origin initially produces a vague, diffuse, aching sensation. Later, as its intensity increases, the pain becomes more localized to the area of the injured organ and is described as more sharp or stabbing.

Visceral pain results from both mechanical and chemical mechanisms: distension, spasm, contraction, stretching, tearing, or ischemia of the gastrointestinal, genitourinary, or other visceral musculature (e.g., heart) or organs (e.g., liver, spleen, pancreas).

Impact of the Undertreatment of Pain

When moderate or severe pain persists for hours, a number of chemical-mechanical feedback loops become established, producing more pain and tissue injury. The results of the undertreatment of severe postoperative pain can range from prolonged convalescence to death.

TABLE 8-2
Factors Affecting the Amount of Postoperative Incisional Pain

Location of Incision

Incisions in the thoracic, upper abdominal, and abdominal regions tend to cause more incisional pain. Transverse incisions of the abdomen generally result in less pain than either vertical or diagonal incisions. Additional mechanical tension on the incision is often responsible for the increased pain.

Size of Incision

Obviously, the more extensive the surgery and incision are, the greater is the incisional pain.

Length of the Procedure

Prolonged exposure and/or retraction of open tissues increases the amount of tissue damage due to traction, stretching, and aeration.

Gastrointestinal inhibition. Uncontrolled pain inhibits gastrointestinal function. Distension caused by decreased gastrointestinal motility causes pain in two different ways: directly by stretching the large bowel and indirectly by increasing tension on the incision in patients who have undergone abdominal surgery. The resulting pain and anxiety cause further release of catecholamines and local pain-producing substances, thereby starting another pain-more-pain feedback cycle, unless the cycle is interrupted by adequate analgesia.

Increased muscle tension. Abnormal muscle contractions result from both reflex muscle spasms and the conscious splinting of painful areas by the patient. For example, after abdominal surgery, a patient naturally consciously splints the incisional area when asked to cough and take a deep breath. After a cough, reflex spasms further increase the voluntary contractions already taking place in the injured muscles. Abnormal muscle tension prevents adequate ventilation of the lungs. Consequently, the amount of retained secretions and the risk of pulmonary complications increase. If ileus also develops, abdominal distension will further decrease the patient's already compromised ventilation by restricting downward movement of the diaphragm.

Persistent pain and the reflex responses after major surgery of the hip, knee, and other major joints can also produce pulmonary dysfunction. The limitation of motion caused by the pain also produces marked impairment of normal muscle metabolism. If the severe pain is allowed to persist, muscle atrophy may occur, prolonging the recovery phase (Bonica, 1982).

Vasospasm. In addition to muscle spasm, uncontrolled pain causes another reflex response, vasospasm, which can result in tissue ischemia. Tissue asphyxia and local acidosis further reduce the pain threshold, triggering another feedback loop: increased pain leading to increased vasospasm, which produces increased pain.

Common complications. The most common postoperative complications associated with the undertreatment of pain, particularly after thoracic and intraabdominal surgery, are atelectasis and pneumonitis. These complications are the result of hypoventilation caused by a combination of involuntary muscle spasm and voluntary splinting of the thoracic and abdominal muscles. Limited movement of the lower extremities increases the risk of thrombus formation. Postoperative patients who restrict their physical activity because they fear creating more pain have a greater prevalence of thrombus formation. Also, heightened anxiety levels in patients with unrelieved pain cause cortically mediated increases in blood viscosity, fibrinolysis, and platelet aggregation, further contributing to the risk that thrombus will develop.

Controlling Postoperative Pain

As alluded to previously, a growing body of literature indicates that relief of postoperative pain is inadequate (Bonica, 1982; Cohen, 1980; Graffam, 1982; Halpern, 1977; Marks & Sacher, 1973). For the most part, this lack of adequate relief occurred because physicians did not order adequate doses of sufficiently potent analgesics. The physicians' actions were then compounded by nurses who tended to administer only 40–50% of the doses ordered (Cohen, 1980; Marks & Sacher, 1973). Consequently, many of the postoperative complications and prolonged disabilities that developed in the past most likely were due to inadequate control of postoperative pain.

Improvements appear to be occurring as a result of increased awareness of the need to improve postoperative pain control and advances in the understanding of pain treatment. New technologies and new applications of old technologies are also contributing greatly to the ability to manage postoperative pain.

Patient-Controlled Analgesia

An important advance has been the development of new methods and routes of drug delivery to maximize pharmacological effects and minimize side effects. Infusion pumps that enable the patient to safely control the frequency of analgesic administration have revolutionized the management of postoperative pain.

The programmable capabilities of the pump allow the clinician to set the size of each increment bolus, to establish the minimum interval between doses, and to lock out any further delivery of medication until the set interval period has expired. A loading dose of analgesic is frequently administered by the nurse rather than by using the pump because the loading dose can be extremely variable. Pharmacokinetics theory suggests that a loading dose hastens the ability to sustain plasma levels of the analgesic at a "pseudosteady state" (Slack & Faut-Callahan, 1991). The major advantage of PCA is that patients have control of their pain management. They do not have to request pain medication and wait for it to be administered. An additional advantage may be that the dose of analgesia can be titrated by administering smaller doses at more frequent intervals. Research has shown that PCA results in better pain control, less total opioid use, and fewer side effects (i.e., improved pulmonary function) than traditionally administered opioid therapy does (Graves, Foster, Batenhorst, Bennett, & Baumann, 1983).

Intraspinal Drug Therapy

Intraspinal delivery of drugs is a powerful method of providing pain relief with minimal side effects. Since its beginning in the 1970s, nurses have been instrumental in managing patients receiving this type of therapy. The major benefit is that it reduces the overall level of opioids required while providing more consistent pain relief. The decreased level of opioids helps prevent the disorientation and oversedation that often accompany parenteral doses. This is especially advantageous for patients in the early postoperative period (Slack & Faut-Callahan, 1991). Patients can become mobile earlier, reducing the risk of complications related to reduced activity.

With this type of therapy, analgesics can be administered in two different ways: intraspinally or epidurally. It is essential that nurses understand the differences between the intraspinal and epidural spaces in order to understand variations in drug absorption and nursing care. Intraspinal spaces are spaces surrounding the spinal cord. The epidural space is the space adjacent to the dural membrane that is composed of adipose and connective tissue and blood vessels. The intrathecal space contains circulating cerebrospinal fluid and is located between the subarachnoid and pial membranes. Both the epidural and the intrathecal spaces are used for safe delivery of medications.

Not all drugs can be delivered intraspinally. Preservatives used in drugs (e.g., alcohol, phenol, and formaldehyde) are toxic to both the central nervous system and the tissue within the epidural space. Therefore, agents administered intrathecally or epidurally are usually preservative-free. Other factors that must be considered are how well the drug is absorbed across membranes and the availability of highly concentrated formulations. Unfortunately, the availability of concentrated, preservative-free drugs, particularly morphine, is limited. New opioids, such as fentanyl and sufentanyl, are approximately 100 and 1,000 times more potent, respectively, than morphine when given intravenously. Intraspinal equianalgesic dosages have not yet been established; however, the intraspinal route may be a useful alternative when patients become tolerant to opioids given by other routes. (Tolerance, a problem in patients with chronic pain, rarely occurs in the acute pain situation.)

Several devices are available for delivering intraspinal medications. These include external catheters, implanted ports, and implanted pumps. External catheters are generally used for postoperative pain. They are also used to deliver anesthetics during surgical procedures. The same catheter may be used for both purposes in a patient.

Safe intraspinal delivery of analgesics requires special care. The catheter in the epidural space can migrate through the dura. It is essential that the nurse be knowledgeable about the pharmacological effect of the drugs being administered epidurally and assess the patient for side effects such as decreased respiratory rate and hypotension. The risk of respiratory depression persists for 6–24 hr after continuous epidural infusion of opioid is stopped (Warfield, 1985).

Use of Potentiators

In many institutions, it is still a common practice to add a so-called potentiator if the first dose of an opioid analgesic does not relieve the patient's pain. Sometimes the dose of opioid is even decreased when the potentiator is added. The potentiator is said to increase the potency of the opioid without increasing respiratory depression or, presumably, the chance of addiction. Unfortunately, the drugs most commonly used as potentiators (Table 8-3) do not actually enhance analgesia.

McCaffery (1982) attributes the popularity of potentiators to the common misconception that a drug that decreases anxiety must automatically lead to decreased pain perception. Pain experts have found nothing to substantiate this belief, however. In one study (Halpern, 1977), for instance, the addition of two aspirin tablets to a regimen of 10 mg of morphine given intramuscularly provided more pain relief than the addition of 25 mg of intramuscular chlorpromazine (Thorazine). Also, McCaffery (1982) notes that the increased sedation that accompanies many of these drugs probably reduces the number of requests patients make for analgesia, not because the patients are comfortable, but because they are too sedated to make the request: "Our willingness to accept sedation and fewer pain reports as evidence of pain relief is possibly a further reflection of our lack of accountability for providing pain relief."

A commonly used potentiator is promethazine (Phenergan). This phenothiazine derivative acts as an antihistamine, an antiemetic, a sedative, and, to some extent, a tranquilizer. Even the manufacturer does not refer to it as a potentiator of opioid analgesia.

The continued use of promethazine as an opioid potentiator is remarkable. For more than 20 years, reports have indicated that it does not add to the analgesia provided by opioids. In a study of postoperative pain, Keats, Telford, and Kurosu (1961) found that promethazine enhanced only the sedative effects of meperidine and did not alter analgesia or respiratory depression. In addition, they did not find any antiemetic effect. Other researchers (Jaffe & Martin, 1975) detected increased respiratory depression. That is, when respiratory depression occurred, it was greater and lasted longer than would be expected with meperidine alone. Furthermore, phenothiazines tend to produce circulatory depression and hypotension. Because they are long-acting drugs, it may take 24–48 hr after their administration before blood pressure is stable enough for the patient to become ambulatory (Halpern, 1977).

Studies have also shown that promethazine is antianalgesic. Doses of 12, 25, or 50 mg of intramuscular promethazine partially blocked the analgesic action of meperidine (Dundee & Moore, 1961). In addition, a dose of 50 mg of intramuscular promethazine alone actually caused an increased sensitivity to somatic pain. These effects lasted approximately 3 hr and were accompanied by a high prevalence of restlessness during the second hour (Dundee, Love, & Moore, 1963).

Factors Determining Administration of Intramuscular Analgesics

Despite all the new advances, for the average patient undergoing major surgery, postoperative pain is managed by intramuscular injections of opioids every 3–4 hr during the first few days after the operation. As mentioned earlier, nurses tend to undermedicate patients postoperatively. The next obvious questions are, How do nurses determine the dose of analgesic and the frequency of administration for individual patients? What criteria do they use to decide who needs more analgesia and who does not? One study looked at this issue (Cohen, 1980). More than 100 nurses were asked to describe the factors they consider when deciding on the dose and time interval for an opioid analgesic for postoperative patients when a flexible dosage and time interval are ordered. The factors they listed are shown in Table 8-4.

Other interesting findings of this study included the following:

● Many nurses (32%) wait for patients to request medication.

● Nurses overestimate the possibility of drug addiction associated with postoperative use of opioid analgesics.

● When given two vignettes in which the only difference was the sex of the patient, nurses se-

TABLE 8-3
Analgesic Properties of Commonly Used "Potentiators"

Agent	Analgesic Action	Comments
Phenergan (promethazine)	Antianalgesic	
Thorazine (chlorpromazine)	Some analgesia	More than one dose may be required to obtain analgesic effect; may be useful in chronic pain to reduce total opioid doses.
Sparine (promazine)	Some analgesia	Same as chlorpromazine, but with less hypotension.
Atarax, Vistaril (hydroxyzine)	Analgesic effect	Partially additive with meperidine and morphine; 100 mg also more effective than 50 mg meperidine given intramuscularly (Stambaugh & Sarajian, 1987). Not as effective orally.
Equanil, Miltown (meprobamate)	Probably none	The perception of pain may be increased by an oral dose of 200–300 mg (Kantor & Steinberg, 1976)
Valium (diazepam)	Unpredictable	Study results are variable. In some subjects, it lowered the pain threshold (Hall, Whitwam, & Morgan, 1974); in some, it increased pain tolerance significantly; and in others, it had the opposite effect (Chapman & Feather, 1984)

TABLE 8-4
Criteria Nurses Use to Determine Use of Parenteral Narcotics in Postoperative Patients

Criteria	% of Nurses Listing this Criteria
Overall size of the patient	52
Type of surgery	36
Severity of pain	34
Time since surgery	32
Response to last medication	28
Age of patient	24
Overall condition and complications	19
Evaluation of vital signs	16
Type of pain	12
Individual pain tolerance	11
Time since last medication	8

selected less medication for pain for female patients.

Nursing Interventions

No new and exciting nursing interventions have been devised to reduce postoperative pain. The mainstays continue to be the appropriate use of analgesics and protection of the patient against unnecessary trauma or traction to the painful regions of the body.

Problem. Fear of coughing or deep breathing.
- Pain source: tension, traction, pressure on incision and injured tissues, compounded by patient's fear of evisceration and pain.

- Nursing interventions
  1. Apply direct pressure to incisional area with pillow, bath blanket, or hands.

  2. Reassure patient that the incision is strong enough to withstand the coughing, and stress the importance of effective coughing and deep breathing.

Problem. Unwillingness to walk or change position or fear of doing so.

- Pain source: tension, traction, pressure on injured tissues compounded by patient's fear of more pain.

- Nursing interventions
  1. Reduce the amount of traction on incision and internal tissues by raising the head of the bed and providing support for affected body parts. Instruct patients how to use of the side of the bed, footstools, and so forth for support when getting out of bed or changing position.

  2. Adequately alleviate patient's pain so that cycle of increasing pain and disability is not established. This may require premedication so that patient's analgesia is at its peak when the patient is turned or walks.

Problem. Abdominal distension.
- Pain source: increased pressure on deep tissues and increased traction on abdominal incision.

- Nursing interventions

1. Prevent the establishment of a feedback loop of increasing pain by using pharmacological and noninvasive methods to relieve pain as soon as possible during the early postoperative period. Use the proper potency of analgesic at the appropriate intervals to avoid unnecessary sedation or undertreatment.

2. Turn the patient and/or have the patient walk regularly to speed the return of bowel motility.

Problem. Excessive anxiety.

- Pain source: patient's anxiety that postoperative pain cannot be controlled.

- Nursing interventions

  1. Assess the level of pain the patient is currently experiencing.

  2. If patient is currently in pain, assess the adequacy of the prescribed and administered analgesia. Administer an appropriate dose or contact physician if orders are not adequate.

  3. Explain (or reexplain) strategies for controlling the pain and the importance of adequate pain control in the prevention of postoperative complications. Do not try to instruct the patient until the pain is controlled.

  4. Instruct the patient about the need to prevent severe pain and how to obtain more analgesia when it is needed.

  5. Discuss the importance of adequately controlling postoperative in order to avoid complications.

OTHER ACUTE PAIN SITUATIONS

Myocardial Infarction

Acute myocardial infarction is often associated with severe, excruciating pain and abnormal reflex responses that may consist of either (1) abnormal vagal function (bradycardia, atrioventricular block, peripheral vasodilatation, and arterial hypotension) that can progress to cardiogenic shock or (2) sympathetic hyperactivity with an increase in cardiac output and myocardial oxygen consumption.

The severe anxiety that invariably develops in patients with acute myocardial infarction further increases these abnormal responses. Moreover, the emotional stress may cause increased blood viscosity and clotting, fibrinolysis, and platelet aggregation, which, as mentioned previously, are potentially dangerous effects of severe anxiety. The combined effect of severe pain is, then, an increased workload for the heart and an increase in its oxygen consumption. If the discrepancy between the oxygen needs of the heart muscle and the available oxygen supply increases, the area of infarction may actually enlarge. Any of these responses may add sufficient stress to the patient's already strained system to cause death. It is therefore critically important that the patient's pain be promptly and adequately relieved.

Studies in animals have shown that interrupting the sympathetic or sensory innervation to the heart can actually reduce the size of an experimentally induced myocardial infarction, reduce the mortality rate, and increase blood flow to the heart muscle (Bonica, 1987). A study of more than 100 patients with severe pain associated with acute myocardial infarction found that a single dose of 0.5 mg of intrathecal morphine provided better pain control than traditional therapy with intramuscular or intravenous opioids. It is not known if patients thus treated have an improved survival rate (Bonica, 1987).

Labor Pain

Bonica (1987) includes labor pain in his discussion of acute pain problems because "although it is the result of a physiologic process, if unrelieved it produces deleterious effects, and also because currently its control is the source of confusion and controversy, and its relief is often refused or outright neglected."

In recent decades, "prepared childbirth" has been the subject of a great deal of enthusiasm. Its strongest proponents have claimed that it can reduce or even eliminate the pain of childbirth. Among these natural childbirth methods (this term has been dropped in recent years) are the following:

● "Childbirth without fear": This was the original program started in 1944 by a physician, Grantly Dick-Read, who thought that pain during childbirth was due to lack of information and anxiety and thus unnecessary.

● The Lamaze method (1970): This program's goal is to produce painless childbirth.

● Sheila Kitzinger's childbirth method (1972): This method uses imagery in conjunction with breathing and relaxation techniques.

● The Bradley method (1974): This method extensively uses imagery and relaxation techniques to reduce pain intensity.

Basically, all these programs include (1) classes that provide detailed information on pregnancy and labor; (2) relaxation training for use during labor and delivery; (3) coping strategies to distract attention from pain; and (4) breathing techniques that are useful in enhancing relaxation, distracting the woman's attention, and aiding delivery.

Despite the claims of these programs, for nearly 8 of 10 women, labor and delivery are associated with moderate to severe or very severe pain. Studies and the experiences of thousands of women have not substantiated the claims that childbirth can be made painless if women are properly prepared for the experience. Melzack et al. (1981) used the McGill-Melzack Pain Questionnaire to measure pain during labor and delivery in 87 primiparas and 54 multiparas. The women were placed in one of two groups: those who received prepared childbirth training and those who did not. The results showed no significant difference in the pain intensity scores between these two groups. "Regardless of the training, the mean [Pain Rating Index score] revealed that labor and delivery pain is amongst the most intense ever experienced by humans" (Melzack et al., 1981). The major values of the preparation appeared to be a more positive and rewarding childbirth experience for any woman who wanted to be actively involved in her labor and delivery and a reduction in the overall amount of anesthesia used by women during delivery because of lessened muscle tension and anxiety.

Studies of primiparas who did not receive medication before labor have shown that the pain of uterine contraction causes a fivefold to 20-fold increase in ventilation, with consequent severe respiratory alkalosis during contractions and hypoventilation between contractions (Bonica, 1987). Common outcomes were fetal hypoxemia and late decelerations of fetal heart rate due to maternal hypoxemia between contractions. Furthermore, as in other acute pain situations, pain and anxiety during labor produce a marked increase in sympathetic activity, with a 50–200% increase in secretion of catecholamine and cortisol and a significant increase in the secretion of corticosteroids and adrenocorticotropic hormone. These chemicals have widespread circulatory effects and cause significant increases in metabolism and oxygen consumption.

If the fetus is normal, it will be able to tolerate the transient impairment of maternal-placental oxygen exchange during contractions. However, if the infant is already compromised because of obstetric or maternal complications, pain-induced reductions in the transfer of oxygen and carbon dioxide may be the critical factors that produce perinatal morbidity, and may even cause death. Studies have shown that adequate relief of pain and anxiety can decrease or eliminate many of the adverse maternal and fetal alterations. Intraspinal anesthetics or analgesics are the safest methods for relieving the severe pain of childbirth. Although intrathecal opioids are useful in relieving labor pain, epidural opioids have not been so successful. A local anesthetic such as bupivacaine, with or without an opioid such as fentanyl, provides adequate pain relief (Bendetti, 1987).

Acute Pancreatitis

Acute pancreatitis causes severe, excruciating pain and severe spasm of the muscles of the abdominal wall and chest, with a consequent decrease in chest wall compliance and an increase in splinting of the diaphragm. It also causes vasoconstriction of the region surrounding the pancreas. This causes the release of toxic substances that depress the cardiovascular system and cause spasms of the duodenum and the sphincter of Oddi. Patients with acute pancreatitis also lose fluid into the retroperitoneal space and peritoneal cavity. All these effects can be sufficient to induce shock. Moreover, the decreased ventilation produces a progressive hypoventilation with increasing hypoxia and hypercapnia. The result can be death. Experience has shown that nerve blocks with local anesthetics or epidural opioids not only provide complete pain relief but also overcome the harmful reflex spasms.

Severe Trauma

In many patients who sustain serious injury, the pain is severe. Their tissue injury and severe pain cause the same reflex changes and anxiety that occur in postoperative patients. Like postoperative pain, severe posttraumatic pain is not always adequately appreciated or relieved. A few studies have shown that block of nociceptive and sympathetic pathways with local anesthetics soon after the injury prevents or promptly eliminates the pain and abnormal reflex responses, with consequent improvement in cardiovas-

cular function. In a critically injured patient, uncontrolled pain can make the difference between life and death.

THE AHCPR GUIDELINE

As mentioned in the introduction to this book, the AHCPR, a division of the U.S. Department of Health and Human Services, has recently published a clinical practice guideline on the management of acute pain. The guideline is designed to help clinicians, patients, and patients' families understand the assessment and treatment of acute pain, including postoperative pain, in adults and children.

Development of the guideline included an extensive literature review to evaluate empirical evidence and significant outcomes. The management model was developed with appropriate linkages. The guideline was drafted and circulated for peer review (which included verbal or written testimony from professional organizations, industry, and patients). It was revised on the basis of the review and then pilot tested. It has been disseminated and evaluated.

Released in February 1992, the guideline is available in several versions to meet different users' needs: *The Clinical Practice Guideline* (includes complete management model with extensive references); *Quick Reference Guide*—versions for pain in adults and pain in children (a summary of information for use in clinical decision making); and *A Patient's Guide*—available in English and Spanish (an informational booklet to increase consumers' knowledge and involvement in health care decision making).

Currently, a group is meeting to determine standards of quality, performance measures, and medical review criteria based on the guideline. It has been speculated that this guideline may be used to determine criteria for reimbursement and accreditation. It is therefore crucial that nurses be aware of and be instrumental in implementing the guideline in the clinical setting.

Copies of the guideline can be obtained by calling the AHCPR Clearinghouse: (800) 358-9295.

SUMMARY

Acute pain and its associated responses are usually the result of tissue-damaging injury or disease. Injury to tissues causes the release of biochemical substances that increase the responsiveness of peripheral pain receptors. Segmental and suprasegmental spinal reflexes and cortical responses lead to systemic changes that cause many of the signs and symptoms characteristic of acute pain. Postoperative pain is of three types: incisional, somatic, and visceral. Inadequate treatment of postoperative pain sets up a feedback loop in which pain leads to more tissue damage, which leads to more pain. The results of undertreatment can range from painful convalescence to death. Other conditions associated with severe acute pain include myocardial infarction, childbirth, acute pancreatitis, and severe trauma.

Methods for controlling postoperative pain include PCA and intraspinal administration of drugs. However, most often, severe postoperative pain is treated by intramuscular administration of opioid analgesics. So-called potentiators do not greatly increase analgesia and may be antianalgesic. Nursing interventions for patients with acute postoperative pain include appropriate use of analgesics and protection against unnecessary trauma or traction to the painful regions of the body.

EXAM QUESTIONS

Chapter 8

Questions 54–64

54. What type of surgery is most likely to cause moderate to severe postoperative pain?

    a. Maxillofacial
    b. Orthopedic
    c. Vaginal
    d. Thoracic

55. In a group of 10 postoperative patients, how many would be expected to complain of pain?

    a. 8
    b. 6
    c. 4
    d. 2

56. Which of the following descriptions most likely refers to incisional pain?

    a. Dull, aching discomfort
    b. Burning sensation
    c. Diffuse, aching sensation
    d. Squeezing sensation

57. Which of the following descriptions most likely refers to somatic pain?

    a. Sharp, cutting pain
    b. Dull, aching discomfort
    c. Burning sensation
    d. Feeling full of pressure

58. Which of the following physiological problems is associated with uncontrolled postoperative pain?

    a. Decreased blood pressure
    b. Tissue ischemia
    c. Increased gastrointestinal motility
    d. Decrease in stroke volume

59. What is a major advantage of the postoperative use of intraspinal opioids?

    a. Increase in overall use of opioids
    b. Better overall kidney function
    c. Faster healing because of earlier mobility
    d. Decrease in the prevalence of central nervous system side effects

60. Which of the following biochemical substances is known to increase the responsiveness of peripheral pain receptors after injury?

    a. Sodium
    b. Magnesium
    c. Potassium
    d. Calcium

61. Studies have shown that nurses tend to administer what percentage of the dosage of analgesic ordered by physicians?

    a. 20–30%
    b. 40–50%
    c. 50–60%
    d. 70–80%

62. In a group of five postoperative patients, how many would be expected to report pain relief when given 10 mg of morphine or less?

    a. 1
    b. 2
    c. 3
    d. 4

63. One advantage of the postoperative use of patient-controlled analgesia is:

    a. Increase in overall use of opioids
    b. Improved pulmonary function
    c. Decrease in opioid-induced nausea
    d. Faster wound healing

64. Which of the following is one of the most common complications of the undertreatment of postoperative pain in patients who have had thoracic or intraabdominal surgery?

    a. Hypotension
    b. Ileus
    c. Atelectasis
    d. Thrombus formation

CHAPTER 9

PAIN IN CHILDREN

CHAPTER OBJECTIVE

After studying this chapter, the reader will be able to describe special pain problems in children, specific approaches used in treatment, and results of studies on pain in this age group.

LEARNING OBJECTIVES

After studying this chapter, the reader will be able to

1. Recognize the results of studies on the amount of postoperative analgesics given to adults compared with the amount given to children.

2. Indicate the drug that decreased metabolic and endocrine stress responses when given to neonates during surgery.

3. Specify one of the most common chronic or intermittent pain problems in children.

4. Specify a dietary treatment that is effective in decreasing recurrent abdominal pain in children.

5. Recognize the results of a study on the relationship between age and sensitivity to pain.

INTRODUCTION

Undertreatment of pain in adults has been well noted, but children with pain are faced with even greater problems. McCaffery (1982) notes that if an adult and a child have essentially the same painful condition (e.g., nephrectomy), "the adult's pain probably will be acknowledged at least to some extent, but the existence of pain in the child may be totally denied or ignored."

Pain control has long been a concern of nurses who care for children. Because of the increasing complexity of care, however, pain management may actually be low on a long list of nursing care priorities. Fortunately, in the past few years, interest in treating children's pain has increased dramatically.

Greater emphasis is also being placed on the essential role nurses play in the assessment and management of pain in children. Many hospitals have sponsored in-service and continuing education programs for nurses on the topic of pain. This chapter provides an overview of the major issues related to control or relief of pain in children.

MYTHS ABOUT PAIN

In addition to the pain myths discussed previously, additional myths about pain in children contribute to the undertreatment of pain in this age group. One myth is that children do not experience as much pain as adults do because the nervous system in children is immature. This statement is open to question, as it is no longer thought that complete myelinization is necessary for the function of nerve tracts. Also, one study (Haslam, 1969) suggests that the younger the child is, the more sensitive he or she will be to pain. Rather than experiencing less pain, children may actually experience more pain than adults.

Another myth is that children recover from painful experiences such as surgery more quickly than adults do. Although children usually are more active sooner than adults after surgery or injury, physical activity is one of the coping techniques children may use to handle unpleasant situations. It cannot be used to indicate the absence of pain.

A third myth is that use of opioid analgesics may cause addiction in children. The prevalence of addiction in adults treated with opioids for pain is extremely low, and there is no reason to expect that psychological dependence (addiction) in children would be any higher.

A fourth myth is that use of opioids in children is dangerous because these drugs cause respiratory depression. If doses are carefully calculated on the basis of body weight, respiratory depression is highly unlikely. Furthermore, the nurse should be closely observing the effect of the initial dose of opioid and then increasing or decreasing the dose according to the degree of pain relief and physiological effects such as respiratory depression. This also makes significant respiratory insufficiency unlikely.

UNDERTREATMENT OF PAIN

Postoperative Pain

One of the most common types of severe acute pain in children is postoperative pain. Unfortunately, available evidence indicates that children receive fewer postoperative analgesics than adults with similar conditions do.

In a group of 170 children, postoperative administration of analgesics was extremely varied in terms of dose and frequency, and many of the children reported moderate to severe pain (Beyer & Levin, 1987). A study (Eland & Anderson, 1977) of 25 children 5–8 years old who were hospitalized for surgery found that 13 children were given no analgesics during the postoperative period. The procedures performed on these 13 children included repair of traumatic amputation of the right foot, excision of a malignant neck mass, and repair of an atrial septal defect. Of the 12 children who did receive analgesics, the number of doses of opioid and/or nonopioid medications ranged from one to five per child. For example, a child with second- and third-degree burns over 65% of the body received one dose of acetaminophen. Only one child received as many as five doses. This child, who had a fractured femur, multiple lacerations, and surgical amputation of the left lower leg, received two doses of codeine and three doses of aspirin. In contrast, a matched-pair study of 18 adults with diagnoses identical to 18 of the children showed that the adults received a total of 372 doses of opioid analgesics and 299 doses of nonopioids, for a total of 671 doses. All 25 children received a total of 24 doses of analgesics.

Other research has shown that, just as in adults, postoperative pain in infants can have worrisome adverse physiological consequences. Anand and Hickey (1987) compared the morbidity and mortality of newborn infants who had undergone ductal ligations with minimal or no anesthesia with that of infants who had received adequate analgesia and anesthesia. Infants who received minimal analgesia had a significant stress response, as shown by a massive outpouring of catecholamines, growth hormone, glucagon, and corticosteroids and a significant suppression of insulin that resulted in prolonged hyperglycemia. Those infants, both premature and full-term, who had received potent analgesia had significantly fewer complications postoperatively and decreased mortality.

Another series of studies examined the stress responses of neonates to surgical trauma. Significant metabolic and endocrine disturbances were discovered in terms of hyperglycemia, glucagon secretion, and insulin suppression, all of which were directly or indirectly attributed to the release of adrenalin. Two groups of premature infants were also tested. One group was given nitrous oxide and curare (extremely light anesthesia). The other was given nitrous oxide, curare, and fentanyl. The differences between the two groups was striking. The endocrine and metabolic stress response was marked in the first group (no fentanyl) and absent in the second group. Moreover, the group that received fentanyl had fewer postoperative complications. The infants who did not receive fentanyl had greater ventilation requirements, more circulatory difficulties, and greater prevalence of metabolic acidosis and intraventricular hemorrhage.

Burn Injuries

Studies have shown that children with extensive burns received significantly fewer narcotics than adults with similar burns did. Attempts have been made to improve pain control for burned children. For example, one center reported that fentanyl, a short-acting potent opioid, was superior to morphine and Percocet (oxycodone plus acetaminophen) for pain relief in children 9–15 years old (Beyer & Levin, 1987).

Burn patients experience both pain and anxiety during dressing changes. These two states must be assessed and managed concurrently by using opioids and benzodiazepines, respectively. As burn dressings are changed repeatedly, tolerance to the opioids and benzodiazepines may develop, necessitating higher doses. The doses should be increased as needed and titrated according to the patient's response. A child may also have ongoing pain. If this pain is not relieved, the child's anxiety during debridement can escalate to a point where large doses of opioids and sedatives will not provide relief. The AHCPR guideline (1992) recommends a continuous infusion or around-the-clock intermittent doses of an opioid and additional bolus doses of an opioid and a benzodiazepine before dressing changes. In addition, for extensive debridement procedures, general anesthesia may be required.

Several nonpharmacological methods have also been tried to improve pain control for children in burn units. One group found that children 7–18 years old who were treated with hypnosis asked for fewer analgesic medications than children in a control group did (Wakeman & Kaplan, 1978). In this study, the children were free to select (within safety limits) the type and amount of medication they received. Unfortunately, no reports of pain intensity were obtained from the children. Thus, it was not possible to determine if pain was actually reduced, because the amount of analgesic medication used may or may not be a valid indicator of pain intensity.

Children as young as 18 months do better during burn dressing changes if their participation and control are maximized (Kavanagh, 1983a, 1983b). For example, the child can help remove the dressings or call for a "time out." Another method of giving control to children is making the time and environment predictable. Dressing changes should take place in a treatment room, allowing the child to consider his or her room a safe place.

Circumcision

A major problem with infants is determining their levels of pain accurately and then relieving the pain safely and effectively. Most research with infants has focused on attempts to describe their responses to pain. Many have targeted observable pain responses and behaviors such as heart rate, crying, body movement or posturing, and facial expression. Some researchers have concluded that facial expressions may be the most consistent indicator of pain in infants (Beyer & Levin, 1987).

Several studies suggest that the acute pain or distress of circumcision or hypospadias repair in male infants and children can be reduced or eliminated by using nerve blocks. Soliman and Tremblay (1978) observed 70 children 4 months to 8 years old during circumcision. Fifty of the children received penile nerve blocks. Of these, only 4% were agitated 15 min after the procedure. Of the 20 who did not receive penile blocks, 90% were agitated. In another study of circumcision pain, 20 infants were given penile anesthetic blocks, and another 19 were not. During the procedure, the infants in the group with the regional block had significantly higher transcutaneous oxygen levels and lower heart rates and cried less than those in the control group. Despite the growing body of literature suggesting the beneficial effects of nerve blocks during circumcision, most are still done without such pain control.

ASSESSMENT OF PAIN

Caring for the child in pain requires frequent assessment and reassessment of the pain, including its presence, amount, quality, and location. Because of the role of emotional distress in pain perception, nurses should explore possible causes of distress and intervene as appropriate. According to the AHCPR guideline (1992), assessment of pain in children should include a pain history (Figure 9-1), a search for diagnoses for the cause of the pain, evaluation of the pain's severity and location, and observation of the child and the child's responses to the environment. Including the parents and other important family members is also crucial. Part of the challenge in treating pain in children is the difficulty of determining the presence of pain and assessing its intensity, particularly in patients too young to express their discomfort verbally.

In general, it appears that the younger the child, the more pain he or she experiences. For example, Zeltzer, Jay, and Fisher (1989) have suggested that the pain of diagnostic procedures is far greater for younger children than for older children because the younger ones are unable to understand the potential long-term benefits of these painful procedures. In some situations, however, developmentally younger children may experience less pain than older children do. This might occur, for example, with pain associated with cancer or juvenile arthritis because the younger children do not associate these diseases with death and disfigurement.

Various pain assessment scales can be used to assess pain in children. The choice of techniques must be based on the child's condition, ethnic and linguistic background, stage of cognitive development, and age. Three approaches are used: self-report, behavioral, and physiological methods. In general, physiological measures are too nonspecific.

Self-report measures are thought to be the most reliable for children more than 4 years old. Scales for children 4–7 years old include simple line drawings of faces; color scales; and the "oucher" scale, which shows pictures of the faces of children with various levels of distress. The adult Visual Analogue Scale can be used in children 7 years and older.

In infants and toddlers, observation and quantification of various behaviors such as facial expressions, posturing, and vocalization or verbalization have been used. Use of behavioral observation to determine pain requires attention to the context of the

Pain Experience History	
Child Form	**Parent Form**
Tell me what pain is.	What word(s) does your child use in regard to pain?
Tell me about the hurt you have had before.	Describe the pain experiences your child has had before.
Do you tell others when you hurt? If yes, who?	Does your child tell you or others when he/she is hurting?
What do you do for yourself when you are hurting?	How do you know when your child is in pain?
What do you want others to do for you when you hurt?	How does your child usually react to pain?
What don't you want others to do for you when you hurt?	What do you do for your child when he/she is hurting?
What helps the most to take your hurt away?	What does your child do for him/herself when he/she is hurting?
Is there anything special that you want me to know about you when you hurt? (If yes, have child describe.)	What works best to decrease or take away your child's pain?
	Is there anything special that you would like me to know about your child and pain? (If yes, describe)

Figure 9-1. Pain history for children. *Source:* U. S. Department of Health.

child's behavior. For example, crying can indicate many things besides pain (e.g., fear, loneliness, overstimulation, or understimulation). The nurse might assume that a child who is sleeping or watching television has no pain, whereas the child may be attempting to control the pain. The Objective Pain Discomfort Scale uses blood pressure, crying, movement, agitation, and verbal report. The CHEOPS (Children's Hospital of Eastern Ontario Pain Scale) scores crying, faces, verbal behavior, position of the torso, touch of the injured area, and the position of the legs. Both of these scales are somewhat complicated to learn and have been validated only in children of certain ages. If care providers are unsure

whether a behavior indicates pain when pain is suspected, a trial dose of an analgesic can be diagnostic as well as therapeutic (AHCPR, 1992).

Multgren (1990) looked at the factors nurses were actually using to determine if postoperative pain was being adequately controlled in critically ill infants. The study showed that the nurses used crying as the major indicator of the presence of pain.

TREATMENT OF ACUTE PAIN

Nearly all approaches used to treat pain in adults can also be used to treat pain in children.

Behavioral Approaches

A number of behavioral techniques have been applied to the treatment of children's pain. These methods can be used independently or in conjunction with analgesic drug therapy.

Children should be prepared before hospitalization, surgery, or painful procedures. Adequate preparation can reduce some of the associated anxiety and thereby reduce the amount of pain experienced. Whenever the child has the ability to understand an explanation, information should be given before the procedure. This explanation should include information about the rationale for the procedure and sensory information about how the procedure may feel. Other preparatory techniques include desensitization, rehearsal, modeling, and hypnosis.

During the procedure, a variety of previously discussed behavioral techniques can be used. Distraction is one of the most effective and widely used. Imaginative techniques can also be used to focus the child's attention away from the present situation and onto something less frightening. When a significantly painful procedure is being performed, pharmacological interventions should be used in conjunction with behavioral approaches.

Hospitalized children often undergo frequent minor invasive procedures, such as finger sticks and venipuncture. These procedures can be a major source of distress. Children will do better if the time and frequency of these procedures are predictable. Therefore clustering the procedures and leaving a block of time that is "safe" is preferable.

Pharmacological Methods

Pharmacological treatment of pain in children should follow the same guidelines used to treat pain in adults. Orders should not call for drugs to be used as needed for pain. The drugs should be selected in order of increasing potency and in a stepwise fashion, and nurses and physicians should regularly assess the level of pain their patients are experiencing.

The management of pain felt by children during painful procedures has been given too low a priority. Spinal taps, bone marrow aspiration and biopsies, incision and drainage of abscesses, bronchoscopy, burn dressing, and suturing are typical procedures performed in children. It is quite clear that lack of attention to pain control during procedures creates a scenario in which each procedure leads to greater fear of the next procedure.

The potent opioid fentanyl citrate is currently being investigated for use in children undergoing painful procedures. The drug is administered transmucosally in the form of a bullet-shaped lollipop. The lollipop is held in the mouth against the buccal mucosa. Adequate levels of the opioid have been achieved with this method. The major advantage is that no intravenous access is needed for analgesia and sedation (Weisman & Schechter, 1991).

Many experts also suggest that an attempt should be made to combine an anxiolytic with an analgesic. Possible choices include combining midazolam with fentanyl or morphine. Alternatively, combining diazepam with either of these opioids would be appropriate (Weisman & Schechter, 1991). Sedation for painful procedures should take place in a treatment room equipped with resuscitative equipment and should be performed by health professionals who are familiar with airway management.

Opioids can be administered to children via the same routes used in adults. The newest technique being widely adopted is PCA. As mentioned earlier, PCA has been used successfully for analgesia in adults.

Preliminary findings indicate that this technique can provide effective relief of postoperative pain in patients 5–18 years old.

Webb, Rodgers, and Stergios (1987) found that children who used PCA used more analgesics during the first 24 hr after surgery than children in a control group but used less thereafter. Over the entire period of analgesic administration, children in the PCA group actually received significantly fewer analgesics and reported greater satisfaction with their pain relief. In a subsequent study, Gureno and Reisinger (1991) reviewed the charts of 15 children who used PCA for relief of postoperative pain. They found that it was a successful method of pain control for children 3 years and older.

Lawria, Forbes, Akhtar, and Morton (1990) reported their experience with PCA in 25 children 5–15 years old. The pumps were loaded with 1 mg/kg of morphine sulfate in 50 ml. A bolus dose of 0.02 mg/kg and a lockout interval of 10 min were the initial settings. The average morphine requirement was 26 μg/kg each hour. Pain control was good with minimal sedation. Adverse effects were few and minor. Education of patients, parents, and nurses was essential for the successful use of PCA. The authors concluded that PCA is an effective and safe means of providing good-quality analgesia in school-age children.

Administration of opioids via epidural or intrathecal catheters is another widely used method for the delivery of these drugs. During surgery, use of an epidural catheter allows the administration of extremely low doses of opioids while avoiding the systemic effects of these agents. In patients with a thoracotomy, an intrapleural catheter can be inserted at the end of the operative procedure. Continuous administration of local anesthetics through these types of catheter has been used successfully in children.

TREATMENT OF CHRONIC AND RECURRENT NONTERMINAL PAIN

Chronic, recurrent pain syndromes are the most prevalent pain conditions in children and adolescents (Beyer & Levin, 1987). The most common chronic or intermittent pain complaints unrelated to serious disease are headaches and recurrent abdominal pain. Serious diseases in which pain is a problem are cancer, hemophilia, sickle cell disease, rheumatoid arthritis, cystic fibrosis, and reflex sympathetic dystrophy.

Nonpharmacological Methods

The effects of a combination of electromyographic biofeedback, relaxation training, and pain behavior management were studied in 20 children 7–12 years old (Beyer & Levin, 1987). The last strategy consisted of having parents reward normal and coping behaviors and discourage maladaptive pain behaviors. Findings showed a significant reduction in duration and intensity of the headaches.

Richter and colleagues randomly assigned 42 children 9–18 years old who had a history of recurrent migraines to two different experimental groups (Richter et al., 1986). Group 1 received relaxation training, and group 2 received training in cognitive control of stress. A third group used as a control received no special training. Compared with subjects in the control group at 1 and 4 months after treatment, subjects in both experimental treatment groups reported less frequent headaches, and those with severe pain reported a significant reduction in pain.

A conservative three-step method for the diagnosis of recurrent abdominal pain in children has been recommended (Beyer & Levin, 1987):

1. Use noninvasive means to rule out organic or psychological causes.

2. Increase dietary fiber.

3. Use more extensive testing to determine the cause of pain.

One well-controlled study examined the effects of increased dietary fiber in 52 children 5–15 years old who had recurrent abdominal pain. Every day for 6 weeks, each child in the experimental group ate two cookies containing a measured amount of corn fiber. The control group received cookies without additional fiber. Children in the experimental group reported fewer attacks of recurrent abdominal pain than those in the control group. This treatment is inexpensive, easy to administer, and may save the child from having to endure more costly and invasive testing or treatment.

The effectiveness of TENS in children has been variable. Some children derive great relief with this method; others do not. Clinicians reported that 60% of the medical-surgical patients seen at the Johns Hopkins Pediatric Treatment Center received adequate relief with TENS (Beyer & Levin, 1987). Randomized controlled clinical trials of this method have not been done with children and are necessary to determine its clinical usefulness in this age group.

Pharmacological Methods

Antidepressants are used to relieve the depression that often accompanies chronic pain conditions, even in children. For enhanced pain control, antidepressants are given in low doses at bedtime. By relieving sleep disturbances and other such problems, these medications help children cope with their pain conditions better and thus manage their lives more positively.

One problem that may contribute to the tendency to withhold injectable opioids from children and infants is the response an injection often produces: a screaming infant or child (McCaffery, 1982). Nurses may think that it is not helpful to cause the child additional pain. However, injections can be set up to help children feel some mastery. They can ge given choices and helped to associate the relief of pain with the injection by having them watch a clock after the injection or by setting a timer. Also, powerful analgesics can safely be given intravenously if an infant or child cannot tolerate oral analgesics. Rectal preparations of opioids are also available. (Oxymorphone suppositories are an alternative to injections of opioids when the oral route is not possible.)

Patient-controlled analgesia is also being used to treat chronic pain in children. Mowbray and Gaukroger (1990) reported their experience with three children who received infusions for up to 41 days. In each case, PCA allowed pain control in difficult situations. In this small series, no tolerance or clinical signs of dependence developed.

Pain Clinics

Adults with chronic pain are often treated in a multidisciplinary pain clinic, and a multitude of treatment approaches are used (see chapter 12). These clinics provide a range of services. Although literally hundreds of pain clinics for adults exist, probably fewer than five clinics in North America are prepared to handle the problems of children with pain (Beyer & Levin, 1987). Suggestions for helping children with recurrent or chronic pain who cannot be treated by a multidisciplinary team include repeated visits to a pediatrician, psychiatrist or psychologist, or nurse specialist with additional training or special insight into children's pain problems. Providing the parents with training guides for teaching their child self-help methods of relaxation may also help.

SUMMARY

Safe and effective techniques are available to decrease the amount of pain a child experiences in an acute care setting. For such techniques to work, however, the pain must be recognized and properly assessed. It should be assumed that anything that will hurt an adult will also hurt a child and that children are, in fact, often more sensitive to hospital procedures than adults are. Assessment and treatment of pain should be a part of every child's care plan. The treatment should be tailored to the child's level of development, physical condition, background, and family situation.

EXAM QUESTIONS

Chapter 9

Questions 65–69

65. Studies on the amount of postoperative analgesics given to adults compared with the amount given to children have shown which of the following?

    a. Adults and children receive equal amounts of opioid analgesics.
    b. Children are given analgesics more frequently than adults are.
    c. Children and adults receive equal amounts of nonopioid analgesics.
    d. Adults are given analgesics more frequently than children are.

66. What drug was shown to decrease metabolic and endocrine stress responses when given to neonates during surgery?

    a. Nitrous oxide
    b. Morphine
    c. Meperidine
    d. Fentanyl

67. Which of the following is one of the most common chronic or intermittent pain problems in children?
    a. Muscular pain
    b. Headaches
    c. Joint aches
    d. Deep bone pain

68. What dietary treatment has been shown to be effective in decreasing recurrent abdominal pain in children?

    a. Decreased lactose
    b. Increased fat
    c. Increased fiber
    d. Decreased sugar

69. What has one study shown about the relationship between age and sensitivity to pain?

    a. The older a person is, the more pain he or she experiences.
    b. The very young and the very old experience less pain than those in other age groups.
    c. Older persons have the same amount of pain as children.
    d. The younger the child is, the more sensitive he or she will be to pain.

CHAPTER 10

MANAGEMENT OF CHRONIC PERIODIC PAIN

CHAPTER OBJECTIVE

After studying this chapter, the reader will be able to recognize mechanisms, signs, symptoms, and treatments of headaches, phantom limb pain, and trigeminal neuralgia.

LEARNING OBJECTIVES

After studying this chapter, the reader will be able to

1. Recognize differentiating features of migraine, tension, and cluster headaches.

2. Indicate some of the major precipitating factors for migraine headaches.

3. Specify drugs that are effective in the control of various types of headaches.

4. Indicate the prevalence of painful phantom limb.

5. Specify current approaches for the treatment of phantom limb pain and trigeminal neuralgia.

INTRODUCTION

Patients with chronic, periodic pain live in a world of uncertainty. One moment, they may feel fine; minutes or a few hours later, they may be overwhelmed by pain. Some patients know what internal or external events can trigger their pain and try to avoid such stimuli. Others have no idea what starts their episodes of pain and feel completely at the mercy of their unpredictable bodies.

Finding tolerable solutions for patients with intermittent pain can be difficult. Their pain is not a symptom of an acute condition that can be reliably eliminated by surgery or some other type of invasive procedure. Also, the pain does not progress relatively quickly, so they do not become impervious to it. Instead, intermittent pain is a useless warning that is out of proportion to the amount of damage that has or is being done to the body. Nevertheless, such so-called benign pain can have adverse effects on a patient's physical and emotional health and the ability to earn a living and on members of the patient's family. Often these intermittent painful conditions are not evaluated or treated aggressively, because the underlying condition is not viewed as potentially fatal. This chapter covers some of the most common periodic, benign painful conditions: recurrent headache syndromes, phantom limb pain, and neuralgias.

HEADACHE SYNDROMES

A person who has never experienced a headache is rare. Headaches are among the most common pain complaints. Americans make more than 50 million visits to physicians' offices and spend more than $400 million on OTC pain relievers each year because of headaches ("Headache," 1987).

Eliminating the pain of an average headache is easy. Usually a couple of aspirins and relaxation are sufficient. However, according to the National Headache Foundation, about 45 million Americans have chronic and recurrent headaches. A recent Harris poll found that this costs U.S. businesses at least $55 million annually in absenteeism and health care costs (Sternbach, 1987).

Because headaches are so common, persons who have recurrent headaches often do not get the attention and emotional support they need from family members, coworkers, or health care professionals. Worse, they are often told that they are causing their own pain. Persons whose lives are severely affected by recurrent headaches are increasingly likely to turn to a clinic that specializes in the problem. These clinics are the reason for the steady improvement in the treatment of headaches. Headache clinics, which offer diagnostic and nondrug and drug therapy, are estimated to help more than 85% of their patients.

The director of the Michigan Headache and Neurological Institute in Ann Arbor reports that 75 percent of patients can bring their headaches under control with the help of drugs, biofeedback, and relaxation tech-

niques. Another 15 percent continue to have headaches but are taught to cope by reducing the need for medication, improving their family relationships and returning to work. "The remaining 10 percent are simply not helpable, and we're not sure why . . ." ("Headache," 1987)

Persons with severe, recurrent headaches consume enormous quantities of analgesics. Many of them eventually become addicted to these drugs. Because of growing tolerance, stronger and stronger analgesics in larger and larger doses are required to keep the pain under control. Their drug use is not limited to analgesics. Tranquilizers and antianxiety drugs such as Valium (diazepam) are also taken in large quantities.

Migraine

Migraine is a recurring headache associated with a group of characteristic signs and symptoms. Migraines can be divided into three major categories:

1. Migraine with aura (classical migraine)

2. Migraine without aura

3. Complicated migraine

Migraine with aura is defined by the International Headache Society (Diamond, 1991) as an "idiopathic, recurring disorder manifesting with attacks of neurological symptoms unequivocally localizable to the cerebral cortex or brain stem, usually developing gradually over 5 to 20 minutes, and usually lasting less than 60 minutes. Headache, nausea, and/or photophobia usually follow the neurological aura symptoms directly or after a free interval of less than one hour. The headache usually lasts 4 to 72 hours."

Migraine headaches do not occur daily. The usual frequency is 1–4 per month. Some patients, however, may have only 1 headache per year, and some will experience as many as 15–16 per month. Some also have cyclic patterns, with cycles lasting 2–20 months and occurring 1–12 times per year.

Auras do not necessarily precede each attack. When they do, the signs and symptoms usually occur 1–2 hr before the headache appears and last less than 1 hr. Approximately 20% of persons who have migraine experience an aura (Freitag & Diamond, 1991). The most frequent signs and symptoms (auras) that may precede classical migraine are as follows (listed in decreasing order of frequency):

- Blind spots (scotomata)
- Bright shimmering or wavy lines (teichopsia)
- Zig-zag patterns (fortification spectra)
- Flashing lights and color (photopsia)
- Paresthesias
- Auditory or olfactory hallucinations

Less common symptoms are hemianopia and illusions of distorted size or shape (metamorphopsia). The distorted figures described by Lewis Carroll in *Through the Looking Glass* (Alice in Wonderland) are thought to be based on the visual distortions he experienced with his migraines.

One patient wrote about her own experience with classical migraines (Didion, 1979):

> Migraine gives some people mild hallucinations, temporarily blinds others, shows up not only as a headache but as a gastrointestinal disturbance, a painful sensitivity to all sensory stimuli, an abrupt overpowering fatigue, a stroke-like aphasia, and a crippling inability to make even the most routine connections. When I am in a migraine aura (for some people the aura lasts fifteen minutes, for others several hours), I will drive through red lights, lose the house keys, spill whatever I am holding, lose the ability to focus my eyes or frame coherent sentences, and generally give the appearance of being

on drugs, or drunk. The actual headache, when it comes, brings with it chills, sweating, nausea, a debility that seems to stretch the very limits of endurance. That no one dies of migraine seems, to someone deep into an attack, an ambiguous blessing.

Migraine without aura is defined as "an idiopathic, recurring headache disorder manifesting in attacks lasting 4 to 72 hours. Typical characteristics of the headache are unilateral location, pulsating quality, moderate or severe intensity, aggravation by routine activity, and association with nausea, photo- and phonophobia."

Patients with migraine without auras may experience premonitions of an impeding attack from 2–72 hours before the headache. The premonitions, which may be vague, include hunger, anorexia, drowsiness, depression, irritability, tension, restlessness, talkativeness, a surge of energy, and a feeling of well-being. These premonitions also can occur in patients with classical migraine (Diamond, 1991).

The headache phase of migraine without aura is usually associated with nausea, vomiting, acute sensitivity to light and sound, and, occasionally, dizziness, fatigue, diarrhea, and light-headedness. The pain is typically on only one side of the head, although it can occur on both sides at the same time and may even switch sides.

The third category of migraine, *complicated migraine*, is characterized by the neurological symptoms that accompany the acute attacks and may persist after the resolution of the headache. These cases can be extremely difficult to diagnose and require extensive testing to rule out cerebral vascular accidents and other types of neurovascular disorders.

Mechanism. Migraine is a complex disorder, and its pathogenesis is still not known. Current research still implicates changes in cerebral blood flow as the major cause of the symptoms (Skyhoj Olsen, 1990).

Precipitating factors. A multitude of environmental factors can trigger a migraine. Stress is the most well-known trigger. Other common factors are foods that contain vasoactive substances such as the following:

- Amines (especially tyramines)
- Caffeine
- Nitrates
- Nicotine
- Monosodium glutamate
- Alcohol

Examples of foods that should be avoided include aged cheeses, pickled foods, fresh-baked yeast breads, marinated foods, bacon, chicken livers, Chinese food, and chocolate.

Nonfood triggers include the following:

- Changes in schedule
- Oversleeping
- Abrupt change in barometric pressure
- Extreme changes in weather
- Flashing light
- Menstrual cycle
- Allergy
- Ringing bell

The following is a story of one woman who was disabled by her severe migraine headaches. It shows how inadequate treatment of migraines can severely reduce the quality of life.

> G.T., age 36, had her first major headache at age 12, with the attacks increasing in severity over the years. "Next to migraines," she told her doctor, the pain of giving birth to her three kids "was a breeze." In 1987 she spent two straight months in bed, incapacitated by pain and nausea. Sometimes the pain was so bad she went to the hospital for shots of morphine. "I had trouble being a mother. My children took care of me instead of me taking care of them." She was taking a wide variety of prescription medications to relieve the pain, but they were doing little good. ("Headache," 1987)

Predisposing factors. The predisposition to migraine appears to be inherited. Diamond (1991) notes that 70% of his migraine patients report a family history of the disorder.

The prevalence of migraines is higher in women (3%) than in men (7%) (Diamond, 1991). For most patients with migraine, the onset of the disorder occurred during adolescence or when they were in their twenties. Remission of migraine usually occurs in the fifth and sixth decades.

Treatment. The outlook for patients with migraine has improved considerably in recent years. Two types of therapies are available. One is aimed at stopping a migraine in progress. The other is used to prevent recurrences.

Preparations containing ergotamine have been used to treat acute migraine episodes for more than 50 years. One review of the literature showed that nearly 80% of patients given ergotamine preparations had complete or partial relief. Ergotamine preparations are classified as vasoconstrictors that specifically counteract the dilatation of some arteries and arterioles, primarily the branches of the external carotid artery.

To be effective, ergotamine must be taken as early as possible in the attack. Patients who have auras should take the drug when the aura occurs. Ergotamine is usually not helpful if it is taken after an attack has been in progress for more than 4 hr.

A common side effect of ergotamine therapy is nausea, which compounds the gastrointestinal complaints associated with migraine. If oral preparations are not tolerated or act too slowly, sublingual preparations may be indicated. Rectal and inhaled preparations are also available. Patients should be carefully taught how to use the particular preparation ordered by their physicians. Rebound phenomena and other problems can develop.

The efficacy of antiinflammatory drugs (NSAIDs) compared with ergotamine preparations is being investigated (Diamond, 1991). In some studies, NSAIDs appeared to be as effective as ergotamines.

When a patient's pain is not adequately relieved by an ergotamine preparation, opioid analgesia may be necessary. Because of the recurrent nature of migraines and the euphoric effect that some patients experience with parenteral opioids, some physicians are wary of using potent analgesics in patients who have migraine.

If a patient has more than two migraines per month, prophylactic therapy should be considered (Diamond, 1991). A variety of therapies are available. Three groups of drugs are now used to prevent migraine attacks (Melzack & Wall, 1983):

1. β-Blockers

2. Antiinflammatories (NSAIDs)

3. Tricyclic antidepressants

Only one drug has received FDA approval for long-term use to prevent migraines: the β-blocker propranolol. This is the drug of choice for preventing migraine (Diamond, 1991). β-Blockers and antiinflammatory drugs prevent headache by their action on blood vessels. Tricyclic antidepressants increase the concentration of norepinephrine and serotonin at the presynaptic neurons in the central nervous system and increase the sensitivity of brain tissue to the action of these two drugs.

Patients should also be taught to avoid, when possible, factors known to trigger their migraines. This may require extensive education about which foods to avoid and about strategies for reducing stress. In some cases, biofeedback has been useful, especially when combined with other techniques (Diamond, 1991).

Cluster Headaches

Few conditions can be mistaken for a cluster headache. These headaches are thought to be the most excruciating of all headaches. They are described as nonthrobbing, boring. They are easily differentiated from migraines. With cluster headaches, the attacks are considerably shorter (30–90 min), always limited to one side of the head (unilateral), occur daily or several times a day, are not throbbing, and are not usually accompanied by nausea or vomiting (Kudrow, 1991). Signs and symptoms associated with attacks are tearing of one eye, rhinorrhea, nasal stuffiness, and redness of the conjunctiva.

According to some physicians, the diagnosis of cluster headaches can almost be made simply by looking at the patient. Most patients are male, smoke tobacco, and have ruddy complexions. During cluster attacks, patients may become violent, rolling around on the ground, hitting their heads against walls, or even jumping out of moving vehicles. They are often thought to be drunk or deranged ("Headache," 1987). They may cry out or scream in desperation. Suicide, although contemplated, is rarely carried out (Kudrow, 1991).

One of the most distressing aspects of these headaches is that they generally occur in clusters. Approximately 80% of patients with cluster headaches have intermittent periods of susceptibility. A period usually lasts for 2 months, with a range of 2–4 months. During this time, a patient may have one to three headaches per day.

An unfortunate 20% of patients have chronic cluster headaches. Chronic cases are characterized by the absence of remission periods for at least 12 months. Furthermore, the frequency of attacks may be greater in chronic types than in episodic cluster headaches.

Mechanism. The underlying mechanism of cluster headaches is unclear. A number of hypotheses have been suggested, but none has been proved.

Treatment. The treatment of cluster headaches includes educating the patient and attempts to prevent further attacks. Patients should be assured that following the prescribed regimen can readily prevent most attacks and taught to treat any that do occur as soon as possible. Patients are also instructed to avoid alcohol, because it may induce an attack. Attacks brought on by travel on airplanes or to high elevation (e.g., mountains) can be prevented by having the patient take acetazolamine daily for 4 days before travel and an ergotamine 1 hr before.

Cluster headaches that occur mainly during sleep can be prevented by taking ergotamine 1–2 hr before bedtime. For attacks that occur during various times of the day or night, other drugs such as methysergide, verapamil, lithium, and prednisone can be used (Kudrow, 1991). In some patients, whiffs of pure oxygen taken when a cluster headache is beginning can relieve the headache just as effectively as a drug can.

Tension Headaches

The most common type of headache is the muscle contraction headache or the so-called tension headache. Certainly, it is the one most widely advertised on television. The pain in this type of headache is typically described as a dull, aching sensation; a tightness or constricting band around the head; or a pressing sensation about the head. Patients often describe their scalp as being too tight, with the feeling that something is swelling and wants to "explode" (Kunkel, 1991). In patients who have a mixed pattern, the pain is often intermittently pulsatile and throbbing, suggesting vascular involvement. The scalp is often tender and sore. Combing the hair may be painful. The neck is often still and tight.

Mechanism. The underlying mechanism of tension headaches is uncertain. Controversy exists as to whether the headache is caused by muscle spasm or is a manifestation of some central neurological mechanism, with the muscle spasm occurring as a secondary phenomenon.

In the past, excessive contraction of muscles around the skull was thought to be the source of tension headaches. This explanation was consistent with the pain and pressure felt by the patient. However, actual measurements of muscle tension have shown no more muscular tightening among patients with tension headaches than among patients with migraine or cluster headaches.

Treatment. The first step in the treatment of tension headache is to rule out other types of headache. This requires obtaining the patient's history and doing a physical examination. After the diagnosis has been established, care must be taken not to turn an intermittent problem into a continuous one. Over-the-counter analgesics are usually sufficient to treat most tension headaches. Some clinicians think that NSAIDs are superior to aspirin, but this has not been proved. None of these medications should be used continuously, however.

The chronic form of tension headaches is often difficult to treat. Because the headache occurs daily or almost daily, patients are often taking daily analgesics and easily become dependent on or habituated to analgesics, tranquilizers, sedatives, and opioids. Caffeine, frequently combined with analgesics, may also cause dependency and perpetuate the ongoing headache.

The medication of choice for chronic (daily or almost daily) tension headache is a tricyclic antidepressant. Nonpharmacological methods used in conjunction with pharmacological treatment are often beneficial. Biofeedback can be helpful in well-motivated patients. Relaxation training and physical therapy can also be useful to loosen up neck and shoulder muscles.

Miscellaneous Headaches

Other types of headaches occur less often than those discussed in the preceding sections but are still troublesome for a great many persons.

Organic headaches. Severe headaches in a person who does not usually have them can be a sign of an organic disorder. The following findings are cause for concern:

● Severe, sudden headaches that seem to come on like a bolt out of the blue

● Recurrent headaches of increasing intensity or frequency

● Headaches accompanied by neck stiffness and fever

● Headaches accompanied by confusion, visual blurring, decreased alertness, sensation, or other neurological deficit

Traumatic headaches. Traumatic headaches are ones that occur after head or neck injury. They may resemble any of the major headache syndromes.

Sex-related headaches. In some persons, headaches are triggered by sexual intercourse. The headache probably is caused by the exertion and the sudden expansion of the blood vessels. In a few persons, severe headache occurs with orgasm. Sex-related headaches usually last about 2 hr. During attacks, ergotamines or antiinflammatories can provide some relief. (Some women report that having sex relieves headache.)

Sinus headaches. Severe sinus congestion or infection can cause a persistent headache that is often confused with migraine or cluster headaches. The treatment is decongestants and, in the case of true sinus infection, antibiotics.

Hangover headaches. Heavy imbibing of alcoholic beverages can result in a severe headache several hours after the drinking stops. This type of headache mimics a migraine and is thought to be a type of withdrawal reaction. Drinking fruit juices with added sugar and other fluids to counteract dehydration can provide some relief. Coffee can also help.

Hunger headaches. Hunger headaches are characterized by a generalized aching of the head, similar to a tension headache. This type of headache is due to going without food for too long.

Temporomandibular joint problems. Temporomandibular joint syndrome affects women more often than it does men. The symptoms may include chronic headaches in the temporal regions. The basic mechanism, and the basis for treatment, is increased jaw clenching during the day and bruxism (teeth grinding) at night. Treatment may include all of the approaches used to treat tension headaches.

Morning headaches. Chronic morning headaches may be a symptom of hypertension or sleep apnea. The patient should have both conditions ruled out.

Summary of Approach to Treating Headaches

The first step in treatment of headaches is to determine their probable source. The next is to treat, whenever possible, the underlying cause. For example, migraine and cluster headaches can be treated with drugs that affect the vascular component of these disorders. Patients with sinus disorders should be treated for the primary sinus condition, not the headache. When headaches are so severe and occur so often that they interfere with the quality of life and require the use of opioid analgesics, muscle relaxants, or other addictive drugs for more than a few days per year, the patient may benefit from referral to a clinic that specializes in the treatment of headaches.

These clinics usually precede any serious treatment with a thorough diagnostic work-up, trying to determine as precisely as possible the type of headache the patient is experiencing. This also enables the clinic to rule out serious organic disorders such as brain tumors. The primary approach to treatment, aside from specific medications for preventing or treating attacks of migraine or cluster headaches, is the same as that used in pain treatment centers not specializing in headaches. The general treatment of patients with chronic pain syndromes and the role of nurses are discussed in chapter 12.

OTHER PERIODIC CHRONIC PAIN SYNDROMES

Phantom Limb Pain

Phantom limb pain is both terrible and fascinating. The prevalence of painful phantom limb is estimated to be between 35% and 67%, depending on how long after surgery the determination is made. For most amputees, the feeling of a phantom limb occurs almost immediately after amputation of an arm or leg (Melzack & Wall, 1983).

> The phantom limb is usually described as having a tingling feeling and a definite shape that resembles the real limb before amputation. It is reported to move through space in much the same way as the normal limb would move when the person walks, sits down, or stretches out on a bed. At first, the phantom limb feels perfectly normal in size and shape—so much so that the amputee may reach out for objects with the phantom hand, or try to get out of bed by stepping on to the floor with the phantom leg. As time passes, however, the phantom limb begins to

change shape. The arm or leg becomes less distinct and may fade away altogether, so that the phantom hand or foot seems to be hanging in mid-air. Sometimes, the limb is slowly "telescoped" into the stump until only the hand or foot remains at the stump tip. (Melzack & Wall, 1983)

The sensation of having a phantom does not require amputation of a body part. Most of us have had local anesthetic blocks for dental procedures that made the anesthetized lip feel bloated. The urge is to constantly touch the lip and inspect it in a mirror.

The phantom is thought to be produced by a lack of nerve impulses from the limb or body area. The central nervous system must sense the lack of normal input. Total blockage of nerve impulses is not necessary, however. The impulses must only be reduced below some critical level. Experiences and observations suggest that the sensation is produced by brain activities that are normally associated with perception of the body's position and image. That is, the mind usually senses the body's position and image from sensory inputs from muscles, skin, and joints. When these inputs are reduced below a critical level, the areas involved in this percepion become spontaneously active so that the limbs are felt in positions that are totally unrelated (in the absence of visual cues) to the position of the real limbs.

The painful phantom. Some amputees have so little pain or feel it so infrequently that they deny having a painful phantom. Others have pains periodically, ranging from several bouts a day to one bout each week or two. A few have continuous pains that vary in quality and intensity. In about 5–10% of amputees, the pain is severe and may become worse over the years. It may be occasional or continuous. It is described as cramping, shooting, burning, or crushing. It may start immediately after amputation, but sometimes it appears weeks, months, or even years later (Melzack & Wall, 1983).

If the pain persists for long periods, other regions of the body may become sensitized so that merely touching these new trigger zones will evoke spasms of severe pain in the phantom limb. Pain may even be triggered by urination and defecation or marked emotional upsets. Surgical procedures patients repeatedly undergo to relieve them of their symptoms often fail.

Treatment. The most effective treatment for phantom limb pain is the injection of a local anesthetic at sensitive spots or nerves in the stump. These blocks can be remarkably effective in stopping the pain for days, weeks, or, sometimes, permanently, even though the anesthesia wears off within hours. Successive blocks may even produce increasingly longer periods of relief (Melzack & Wall, 1983).

Lumbar epidural blocks (with both a local anesthetic and morphine) 72 hr before surgery reduce the prevalence of phantom limb pain. Table 10-1 shows the striking results of using a preoperative regional block before amputation. The explanation for the results is that the anesthetized tissues cannot transmit electrical impulses. Thus, repeated barrages of pain impulses from the limb before and during surgery do not reach the spinal cord. Studies in animal have shown that when the spinal cord receives a barrage of pain impulses, a widespread hyperexcitability is triggered. It is hypothesized, then, that if the cord hyperexcitability is allowed to subside by giving the spinal cord a 3-day rest before surgery and then blocking massive inputs of noxious stimuli during the amputation itself, phantom limb pain is less likely to be started. If it does occur, it is less likely to become a chronic problem.

Phantom body pain in paraplegics. Phantom body pain in paraplegics is one of the most mysterious of all pain phenomena (Melzack & Wall, 1983). Immediately after severe damage to the spinal cord, a person may have no sensation below a certain level of the body, the level of the spinal damage. Sometimes, even though stretched out straight on the bed, the legs feel as if they are up in the air with the toes over the head.

Paraplegic patients report three types of pain:

1. Root pain localized at or near the level of the lesion in the spinal cord

2. Visceral pain that usually accompanies a distended bladder or bowel

3. Phantom body pain that is felt in the areas of complete sensory loss

---

TABLE 10-1
Number of Patients Experiencing Phantom Limb pain

Procedure Used	Time After Surgery		
	7 Days	6 Months	1 Year
No preoperative block (14 patients)	9	5	3
Lumbar epidural block started 3 days preoperatively (11 patients)	3	0	0

Source: Bach, Noreng, & Tjellden, 1988.

It is estimated that 5–10% of paraplegic patients have severe phantom body pains. The patients complain of burning, tingling pains in segments of the body below the level of the lesion, segments in which they have a complete loss of sensation to sensory stimuli. These pains are sometimes replaced by a sensation of severe, crushing pressure; vicelike pinching sensations; the feeling that streams of fire are running down the legs into the feet and out the toes; or by a pain that feels as if a knife is being buried in the tissue, twisted around rapidly, and finally withdrawn, all at the same time (Melzack & Wall, 1983). The pain may start immediately or occur months or years after injury. In a few patients, the pain persists for years without abating and leads to multiple operations: rhizotomies, cordotomies, and sympathectomies. Most of these operations do not provide lasting relief.

The pain felt by these patients resembles phantom limb pain, and the neural mechanisms may be similar. In paraplegics, even more so than in amputees, the loss of sensory input to cells in the spinal cord below the level of the lesion is enormous. This loss appears to produce highly abnormal activity in these cells. Although phantom limb pain can now be helped in a significant proportion of amputees by reducing the inputs to the spinal cord (Bach, Noreng, & Tjellden, 1988), the pains suffered by paraplegics are less easily treated (Melzack & Wall, 1983).

Neuralgias

Several pain syndromes associated with peripheral nerve damage are generally categorized as neuralgic pain. They are similar to phantom limb pain and are characterized by severe, unremitting pain, which is difficult to treat. The causes of neuralgic pain include viral infections of nerves, nerve degeneration associated with diabetes, poor circulation in the limbs, vitamin deficiencies, and ingestion of poisonous substances such as arsenic. In brief, almost any infection or disease that produces damage to peripheral nerves, particularly the large myelinated nerve fibers, may be the cause of pain that is labeled as neuralgic.

Trigeminal neuralgia, also called tic douloureux, almost always begins after the age of 30 years. Exceptions are patients with multiple sclerosis, in whom it can occur at any age. The pain is intense and occurs in association with trigger zones (areas of increased sensitivity on the face). The pain can be set off by the lightest touch or sensation. Patients with this condition often avoid touching, washing, or shaving the face; biting; and chewing. Knowledge of this avoidance is valuable in making the diagnosis. In almost any other type of facial pain, patients massage the affected area.

The pain is paroxysmal and usually lasts less than 20–30 sec. This is followed at times by a period of relief that lasts for a few seconds to a minute and then another jab of pain. Repeated episodes of pain may occur, but the pain is not long-lived as other chronic facial pains (Dalessio, 1991).

Similar patterns of pain (with trigger zones and short-lived intense pain) in areas of the body supplied by other nerves are being recognized more often in patients with multiple sclerosis. These are treated in the same manner as trigeminal neuralgias.

Treatment. Both medical and surgical therapies may be used in the treatment of trigeminal and other neuralgias. Ordinarily, the treatment is medical. However, if the pain is not relieved by drugs, or if the patient has a toxic reaction while taking medications, surgical interventions may be needed. The drugs used initially are anticonvulsants, such as carbamazepine (Tegretol). Selective lesions of the nerve root can be created by using a radio-frequency electrode (radio-frequency rhizotomy) in a surgical procedure. This procedure is safe and simple and effective in 90% of cases. The recurrence rate in trigeminal neuralgia is about 25%, however. Newer procedures and medications are being tested at centers throughout the United States.

EXAM QUESTIONS

Chapter 10

Questions 70–80

70. Which of the following foods is most likely to precipitate a migraine headache?

    a. Milk
    b. Alcohol
    c. Sugar
    d. Beef

71. What is the prevalence of phantom limb pain?

    a. 3–18%
    b. 20–32%
    c. 35–67%
    d. 70–89%

72. What type of headache is sometimes described as a throbbing pain on one side of the head preceded by an aura?

    a. Tension
    b. Sinus
    c. Hunger
    d. Migraine

73. Which of the following drugs has been effective in the treatment of trigeminal neuralgia?

    a. Lithium
    b. Carbamazepine
    c. Valium
    d. Thorazine

74. What type of drug has been successful in preventing migraines?

    a. Opioids
    b. β-Blockers
    c. Antihistamines
    d. Vasodilators

75. What type of headache is associated with nausea and vomiting, sensitivity to light, and occasional dizziness?

    a. Organic
    b. Migraine
    c. Temporomandibular
    d. Sinus

76. Which of the following has been most effective in the treatment of phantom limb pain?

    a. Intrathecal opioids
    b. Transcutaneous electrical nerve stimulation
    c. Biofeedback and relaxation techniques
    d. Local anesthetic to the stump

77. What type of headache is usually described as a dull, constricting ache on both sides of the head?

    a. Tension
    b. Cluster
    c. Hunger
    d. Migraine

78. What is the drug of choice for treatment of chronic tension headaches?

    a. Opioids
    b. β-Blockers
    c. Tricyclic antidepressants
    d. Muscle relaxants

79. What type of headache nearly always occurs on one side of the head with an intense, stabbing pain near the eye, which frequently drips tears?

    a. Tension
    b. Cluster
    c. Sinus
    d. Migraine

80. Which of the following drugs has been effective in the prevention of cluster headaches?

    a. Morphine
    b. Thorazine
    c. Valium
    d. Lithium

CHAPTER 11

MANAGEMENT OF CANCER PAIN

CHAPTER OBJECTIVE

After studying this chapter, the reader will be able to recognize sources, severity, management techniques, and treatment of pain associated with cancer.

LEARNING OBJECTIVES

After studying this chapter, the reader will be able to

1. Specify the percentage of cancer patients with advanced stages of disease who experience pain.

2. Recognize the pain syndromes associated with use of vinca alkaloids in the treatment of cancer.

3. Specify how patients in severe and chronic pain are likely to react when asked to describe their pain.

4. Specify a major innovation for managing moderate to severe pain.

5. Differentiate between the timing of peak plasma levels of oral and parenterally administered doses of morphine.

6. Specify the side effect that has been associated with the use of intraspinal opioids.

7. Select the tranquilizer that has been most effective in the treatment of prolonged pain.

8. Recognize the earliest sign that tolerance is developing to an opioid.

9. Indicate a coanalgesic by its mechanism of action.

10. Specify the type of coanalgesic useful in the treatment of pain associated with bony metastases.

INTRODUCTION

It is a common belief among members of the public that cancer and pain are invariably linked. Persons experiencing persistent pain almost immediately become concerned that the pain may be a symptom of cancer. Certainly, most think that a person dying from cancer is always in severe pain.

What actually is the relationship between cancer and pain? This question has no simple answer. The following statistics indicate the prevalence of pain in various stages of this disease (Twycross, 1985):

- Nonmetastatic cancer: 15%
- Metastatic cancer: 33%
- Advanced stage of disease: 60–90%

For cancer patients and their care providers, the most relevant statistics are the ones that indicate that large numbers of cancer patients die without relief from severe pain (Twycross, 1985). One study estimated that 25% of all patients with cancer throughout the world die in severe pain. Despite numerous advances in the treatment of cancer pain, patients continue to suffer needlessly. The reason is deficient understanding of the principles of pain management in terminal disease (Bonica, 1987; Foley, 1985; Lipman, 1980; Mount, 1984; Twycross, 1985). This chapter discusses current management guidelines for patients with pain due to cancer.

THE EFFECTS OF UNDERTREATMENT OF PAIN

The belief that undertreatment of pain is not as serious as undertreatment of disease, particularly in cancer patients, continues to persist. Only recently have health care providers recognized that pain itself can be destructive to the patient.

Physical and Psychological Effects

Usually the physiological and psychological effects of pain due to cancer are greater than those of chronic pain unrelated to cancer. The physical deterioration is more severe because cancer patients have greater problems with sleep disturbance, nausea, vomiting, and lack of appetite. They also have more emotional reactions such as anxiety, depression, hypochondriasis, a tendency to focus on their symptoms, and neuroticism in response to pain (Figure 11-1).

Overwhelming Pain

After months of severe pain, particularly if it is associated with insomnia, some cancer patients become overwhelmed with the pain. They often find it difficult to describe the location or the nature of the pain precisely. They may say, "The pain is in my chest, my back, my arm—it's everywhere." In most cases, the patient becomes mentally and physically withdrawn.

Bill was a well-known composer in his midthirties who had multiple myeloma. By the time a pain specialist met him in the hospital, he lay in his bed for days on end, not speaking to his wife or parents and not eating. He barely responded when the specialist

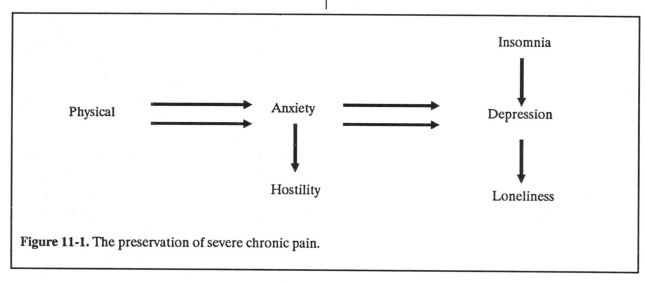

Figure 11-1. The preservation of severe chronic pain.

introduced herself and asked him a few questions. He looked and acted severely depressed. Finally, she said to him, "How bad is your pain?" He looked at her for the first time. With no emotion in his face, he said in a quiet voice, "It is bad enough that if it does not get better in the next week, I am going to kill myself."

Bill's physicians and nurses were unaware of his severe pain. He did not writhe in agony, and he did not ring his bell constantly asking for more medication. Bill had given up hope that his pain could be controlled with medication, so he did not think it was worthwhile trying to convince his health team that he was overwhelmed with pain. His only hope was that the chemotherapy would reduce the pain by shrinking his tumors.

A subgroup of patients with overwhelming pain do not exhibit vegetative behaviors. In these patients, usually those whose pain is exacerbated by movement, marked anxiety is the prominent symptom. They tend to fear any movement or being moved, are persistently anxious and agitated, and generally have no faith in any pain medication. Some have a mixture of depressive and agitated features (Lack, 1984a).

Anxiety can be a problem in cancer patients even when pain is not a major symptom. Still, overwhelming pain is certainly a rational reason for becoming extraordinarily anxious. Even when marked anxiety is present, however, it is not always readily apparent. In such instances, the health team should look for behaviors such as the following (Lack, 1984a):

● Attention-seeking behaviors
● Fear of being left alone
● Hyperactivity
● Unpleasant or frightening hallucinations
● Nightmares
● Continued insomnia despite pain relief

Patients with overwhelming pain can be difficult for the nursing staff to help, as shown in the following case:

Mary was a professor from a local university. In her late fifties, she took a straightforward approach to her cancer and cancer therapy. She had never married, and her parents, both in their eighties, were her only relatives. Now in the final stages of her disease, Mary had been having uncontrolled pain. It was under better control after a week in the hospital, but Mary was extremely anxious and very demanding of her parents and staff personnel. Whenever her family left in the late afternoon, she constantly rang her bell or yelled to get the staff members' attention. Antianxiety agents, frequent visits by nurses, and psychological intervention were not effective in relieving Mary's severe anxiety. Eventually, nonprofessional attendants were hired at the parents' expense to stay with Mary at night during her last weeks. Only then did the terrifying anxieties leave and allow her to have some peace of mind.

Although Mary probably had unresolved psychological issues that led to her persistent terror of being alone, she was unable to deal with them as death approached. She probably would have felt less isolated if she had not been in a private room with no contact with others for many hours at a time.

Private rooms, in which terminal patients are usually placed, effectively isolate patients who do not have someone who can stay with them, particularly at night. This is usually not the case in English hospices, which are the source of much of what is known about how to care for patients who are in pain or terminally ill. In English hospices (and hospitals), patients are much more likely to be in a ward with other patients.

Being on a ward has drawbacks, such as lack of privacy, but at least patients are not totally alone, with little interaction with others to provide distractions from pain and fear. Sometimes, simply listening to staff members talk or talking with patients in adjacent beds or with someone else's visitors can help. This is often preferable to lying alone in a room with nothing except the television.

Members of the hospital staff can counteract the isolation inherent in private rooms. Intermittent visits to a patient's room when the patient is alone, proper use of analgesic and antianxiety medications, and discussions with patients about their concerns and fears are all important ways to help patients overcome the sense of isolation. In some facilities, the health team's efforts are supported by specially trained volunteers who are available to sit with highly anxious patients. Ideally, this service would be available in all acute care facilities.

Outcome of Undertreated, Chronic Pain

Eventually, persistent, severe pain leads to invalidism, and the patient often becomes bedridden. The resulting decalcification of the bones, muscle atrophy, and perhaps even contractures further contribute to the patient's debilitation. Poor nutritional intake leads to protein and vitamin deficiencies, which increase the general debilitation taking place. The patient's cognitive processes slow because of depression and the absence of normal mental stimulation. The patient becomes terminal, not because of the underlying disease but because of the inadequate management of severe pain.

INADEQUATE TREATMENT OF CANCER-RELATED PAIN

Patients with pain related to cancer often have concomitant psychological and emotional pain as a consequence of the diagnosis itself. They require the most sophisticated pain treatment the health team can provide. However, as discussed in the introduction to this chapter, many thousands of cancer patients still die with unrelieved pain. Why is their pain unrelieved?

Inadequate pain relief in cancer is rarely due to the lack of available means for controlling it. Rather, it is usually the result of deficiencies on the part of the health team, the patient, and the patient's immediate family.

Common Reasons for Unrelieved Pain in Cancer Patients

A television call-in show featured a discussion on legalizing heroin in the United States so the drug could be used to treat severe pain in the terminally ill. The station was deluged with calls from families telling horrific tales of the unrelieved agony they witnessed when a loved one was dying from cancer. Many related being told similar excuses by physicians: "Nothing more can be done. We're using the strongest medications we have, and they aren't strong enough."

Although these callers were mistaken about the supposed superiority of heroin for the treatment of pain, their experiences suggest that many health care teams do not adequately use the resources that are available for treatment of severe cancer pain. In this day and age, a terminal patient's severe pain should never be judged uncontrollable.

Many reasons account for the inadequate treatment of pain in cancer patients, but the lack of sufficiently potent drugs is not one of them. Twycross, a surgeon and cancer pain specialist in England, outlined the problems he encountered most often in his practice (Twycross, 1978). Many are similar to those found in clinical settings throughout the United States. The following sections outline his findings and supplement them with additions specific to hospitals in the United States.

Fault with Actions Taken by the Patient or the Patient's Family

1. The patient does not inform the health team about the true severity of pain problems because the patient thinks that pain is inevitable and untreatable in cancer or because the patient tries to "put on a brave face."

2. The patient is not actually taking the analgesics prescribed by the physician:

   - The patient does not believe in taking pain medications.

   - A prescribed analgesic caused troublesome side effects, so the patient stopped taking it and did inform the health team.

3. The patient does not comply with instructions on how to take potent analgesics:

   - The patient thinks that analgesics should be taken only when "absolutely necessary."

   - The patient or the patient's family fears addiction if opioid analgesics are taken regularly.

   - The patient thinks that tolerance will develop rapidly, leaving nothing "for when things get really bad."

Fault with the Health Team

1. The severity of the pain is not appreciated because of inadequate questioning of the patient and inadequate assessment of the patient's symptoms and situation.

2. Prescription and/or administration of analgesics is improper.

   - The analgesic prescribed is too weak to relieve much or any of the patient's pain.

   - The prescribed dose of a potent analgesic is too low because the health team is not aware that standard drug doses (derived from postoperative studies) have no relevance in the management of cancer pain, particularly in patients who have been on opioid analgesics for some time.

   - Because of a lack of knowledge about equianalgesic doses, the physician either reduces or does not increase the dose of analgesic when switching from one preparation to another.

   - The team fears that the patient will become addicted if an opioid analgesic is administered regularly.

   - Side effects associated with the use of opioids are not adequately recognized and treated (or prevented).

   - The team thinks that morphine and other potent opioid analgesics should be reserved until the patient is "really terminal" (i.e., moribund).

   - Analgesics are prescribed to be used as needed for pain rather than on a regular basis for patients with persistent pain.

- A prolonged-release morphine tablet is cut up, a step that destroys the tablet's prolonged action.

- Instructions to the patient about optimal use of the prescribed analgesic are inadequate.

- The patient's response to pain interventions is not monitored adequately.

- Coanalgesics, other drugs, or noninvasive techniques are not used in conjunction with analgesics in order to enhance overall pain relief without increasing side effects.

- The informational and emotional support given to the patient and the patient's family is inadequate.

3. The deleterious effects of prolonged, unrelieved pain on patients' health and wellbeing are not recognized.

Finally, neither nurses nor physicians are held responsible if their treatment plan does not control a patient's pain. In addition, careful reassessment of what treatment has actually been given and at what intervals, the patient's responses, and so forth is seldom done. Instead, random, often irrational, changes in analgesic drugs, doses, and administration intervals are tried. Unfortunately, despite their lack of expertise, oncologists and general surgeons in many institutions do not seek advice from specialists in pain management (Twycross, 1978).

Mechanisms of Pain in Cancer

Cancer patients may have pain for a number of reasons, depending on the location of the tumor, the stage of disease, and each patient's pain threshold. Pain due to cancer has a variety of causes:

- Pressure on a nerve caused by the tumor (nerve compression)

- Ulceration with or without the presence of infection or inflammation

- Impaired circulation due to blocked vessels

- Blockage of an organ

- Malignant bone lesions with or without muscle spasm

- Tumor infiltration of soft tissues

Furthermore, pain disorders related to the cancer treatments, not the cancer itself, may develop. The following list gives examples of these treatment-related disorders:

- Postoperative neuralgias
- Postchemotherapy neuropathy
- Postradiation fibrosis or myelopathy
- Phantom limb pain

Among cancer patients with pain seen at Memorial Sloan-Kettering Cancer Center, pain was due tumor involvement in nearly 8 of 10 patients (78%). Half of these (39%) were due to metastatic bone disease, one fifth (19%) to nerve compression or infiltration, and only a small number to involvement of a hollow viscus. Pain caused by cancer therapy accounted for the pain complaints of approximately 1 in 5 patients (19%) (Foley, 1985).

These findings are consistent with reports from other institutions. Of the different types of pain, bone pain was said to be most resistant to pain therapy. An interesting finding was that patients' descriptions of their pain differed according the physical basis of the pain:

- Throbbing: bone lesions
- Aching: nerve involvement

- Sharp: soft-tissue pain
- Tender and burning: treatment-related pain

Postoperative Pain Syndromes

The common feature of postoperative pain syndromes is pain due to interruption of sensory nerves during a curative or palliative surgical procedure. The pain usually begins 4–6 weeks after the procedure, at the time when incisional pain is clearing. An acute piercing pain occurs first and then appears to dissolve into a second type of pain, a burning dysesthetic or hyperesthetic pain in an area of sensory loss caused by the surgery. The pain is associated with a sensation of constriction or tightness in the area of sensory loss. Specific syndromes include pain after mastectomy or thoracotomy and phantom limb pain (Foley, 1985).

Pain after mastectomy. Pain after mastectomy is felt in the posterior part of the arm, the axilla, and the anterior part of the chest wall 4–6 weeks after surgery. It appears to be caused by interruption of the intercostobrachial nerve. This syndrome appears most commonly in patients who have severe local swelling or infection after radical mastectomy.

Pain after thoracotomy. In a small percentage of patients who have thoracotomy, pain occurs along the distribution of an intercostobrachial nerve after surgical injury. Movement exacerbates the pain, and a frozen shoulder may develop.

Pain after amputation. Pain after amputation is of two types: stump pain and phantom limb pain. New data show that use of a continuous regional block in the limb to be amputated, starting 3 days before surgery, may prevent phantom limb pain from becoming a chronic problem (Bach et al., 1988).

Pain Syndromes Associated with Chemotherapy

Several pain problems occur during or in association with chemotherapy.

Peripheral neuropathy. Peripheral neuropathy is a side effect of certain widely used chemotherapeutic agents known as vinca alkaloids. The syndrome starts as a tingling in the extremities after several treatments with these drugs. Rarely, the symptoms may progress to a chronic pain problem with peripheral neuropathy.

Pseudorheumatism. Both rapid and slow withdrawal of high doses of corticosteroid medications in patients taking these drugs for either short or long periods is associated with pseudorheumatism. The syndrome consists of diffuse myalgias and arthralgias, with muscle and joint tenderness on palpation but without objective signs of inflammation. A sense of general malaise and fatigue is common. Signs and symptoms revert with reinstitution of corticosteroid treatment.

Aseptic necrosis of bone. Aseptic necrosis of bone is a complication of long-term treatment with corticosteroids. The heads of the humerus and femur are affected most often. Pain in the shoulder or knee and leg is a common complaint. Radiologic evidence of change is not detected for several weeks to months after the onset of pain.

Pain Syndromes Associated with Radiation Therapy

Radiation fibrosis of a major nerve plexus. Fibrosis of the brachial nerve plexus is associated with irradiation of the chest and upper part of the arm. Fibrosis of the lumbar plexus may occur after irradiation of the lower part of the spine.

Radiation necrosis of bone. The signs and symptoms of radiation necrosis of bone are similar to those of necrosis caused by prolonged treatment with corticosteroids. Most commonly, the heads of the humerus and femur become necrotic after irradiation of the shoulder or hip, respectively.

Pain Unrelated to Cancer or Cancer Therapy

A common misconception is that pain in patients with cancer is always directly related to the tumor.

This is not true. Patients with cancer are as prone (if not more so) to other types of painful conditions as other persons of the same age and sex are. Examples are the pain of arthritis, tension headaches, musculo-skeletal disorders, and cystitis (Twycross, 1985).

Health professionals should be aware that terminally ill cancer patients typically have more than one pain. In one study of cancer patients with pain in more than one site, about half the patients had some pain caused by their cancer and some pain associated with nonmalignant diseases (Twycross, 1985).

TREATMENT OPTIONS

Several strategies can be used to treat pain in patients with cancer. Some are limited to patients in advanced stages of disease who have no hope of cure. Others can be used for patients in all stages of disease. The four primary approaches are as follows:

1. Those that modify the pathological process

2. Those that affect the perception of pain

3. Those that raise the pain threshold

4. Those that reduce the production of pain

Optimal pain control may require a combination of two or more approaches.

Modifying the Pathological Process

Nearly all approaches used to cure cancer can also be used to treat pain due to cancer. These treatments are used in advanced stages of disease to reduce the size of the tumor or tumors and thus directly reduce pain caused by tumor pressure or infiltration.

Radiation therapy. Radiation decreases the pain caused by a variety of malignant tumors. It is most effective and is used most frequently in patients with metastatic bone tumors. The metastatic bone lesions most sensitive to radiation are those from breast cancer. Local irradiation of the tumors provides pain relief in 70–80% of patients. It also helps promote new bone formation and thus prevents pathological fractures. Radiation is also effective for osseous lesions from metastatic bronchogenic, thyroid, and kidney cancers and for prostatic lesions in the pelvis (Foley, 1985).

Other malignant conditions for which noncurative radiation therapy is used for pain control are head and neck cancers; brain tumors; lesions of the brachial plexus; and obstructive lesions of the kidney, bowel, and genitourinary tract.

Chemotherapy. Chemotherapy is sometimes used to provide pain relief when a patient has no chance of cure or even of significant prolongation of life. Sometimes tumors are in body locations where radiation cannot be safely used. In other cases, the tumors are so widespread that radiation is not possible. In these situations, systemic chemotherapy is the treatment of choice. For example, although radiation therapy is effective in cases of bone metastases from breast and prostatic cancers, systemic chemotherapy with hormones or other agents can treat all lesions simultaneously. When tumors highly resistant to chemotherapy and radiation therapy are localized in certain body regions (e.g., advanced stages of head and neck cancer), high doses of chemotherapeutic agents may be perfused locally to relieve pain without causing excessive systemic toxic effects. The tumor, although resistant, often is affected by the extremely high doses used locally.

Antiinflammatory drugs. Antiinflammatory drugs reduce pain by reducing inflammation, which is an alteration of the pathological process.

Surgery. Surgery can be useful in a number of distressing problems caused by advanced stages of cancer. For example, a simple mastectomy may be performed in a woman with an advanced stage of breast cancer both to alleviate discomfort caused by the ulcerated breast and to eliminate problems posed by the draining breast lesion. In other cases, surgery may be used as a comfort measure to relieve obstruction caused by metastatic lesions in the terminally ill. And finally, the most frequent use of surgery in advanced stages of cancer is to alter the patient's hormonal status. Examples are removal of the ovaries in premenopausal females with estrogen-positive breast cancer and removal of the testes in males with prostatic cancer.

Altering the Perception of Pain

Treatments to alter the perception of pain include all of the following (see chapter 5 for details):

- Opioid analgesics
- Neurosurgery
- Regional blocks
- Acupuncture
- Distraction
- Skin stimulation
- TENS
- Counterirritants
- Hypnosis
- Guided imagery
- Biofeedback

Use of pharmacological agents is by far the most frequent method of treating pain related to cancer. In part, this is because both patients and health care professionals have confidence in the ability of drugs to relieve pain. Also, use of analgesics does not require a highly sophisticated health team to initiate treatment or monitor administration.

Raising the Pain Threshold

A person's pain threshold is raised by altering factors known to positively or negatively affect it. That is, the health team attempts to remove or reduce factors that lower a patient's threshold to feeling pain and to increase factors that raise the threshold (Table 11-1).

Reducing the Production of Pain

Pain can also be relieved (or at least markedly reduced) by reducing or eliminating the production of noxious stimuli by the malignant lesions or accompanying disorders. This differs from the first approach because the pathological process itself is not being affected. For example, with this approach, a patient with multiple malignant bone lesions would be placed on an air bed so that turning is not necessary. This will not affect the progression of disease, but it will reduce the pain produced by turning the patient. Or, if a patient has a solitary pathological fracture in the arm, immobilization of the affected area in a sling could greatly reduce the pain while radiation or chemotherapy is under way.

ASSESSMENT OF PAIN RELATED TO CANCER

The initial step in the treatment of pain in a patient with cancer, whether in the inpatient, outpatient, or home setting, is the same as that for any patient complaining of pain: an assessment of the pain. When a patient has been in severe pain for some time, the assessment often must wait until the pain has been controlled with analgesics for several days.

Cancer patients also tire easily, especially those with chronic pain. The health team needs to be sensitive to the patient's physical and emotional state. Sometimes close family members can answer questions, thus reducing the number of questions put to the

Table 11-1
Factors That Alter the Pain Threshold

Lower Threshold	Raise Threshold
Insomnia	Relief of symptoms
Fatigue	Sleep
Anxiety	Emotional support
Fear	Relaxation
Anger	Increased understanding
Sadness	Laughter
Isolation	Social interactions
	Analgesics
	Antianxiety agents
	Antidepressants

patient. For example, the spouse can often give exact details about the patient's medications, doses, treatments, and so forth.

Several questions should be asked about the pain. The health care team can use the patient's answers to (1) develop a plan for maximizing analgesic effectiveness, avoiding pain-inducing factors, and enhancing pain-relieving interventions and (2) establish a baseline for judging the effectiveness of pain-relief interventions in the future.

What Does the Pain Feel Like?

What words does the patient use to describe the pain? Nurses should keep in mind that patients in severe, chronic pain may have difficulty answering many of these questions. They should not assume that an inability to be precise indicates that the pain is being exaggerated. Also, many patients have difficulty describing their sensations. It may be necessary to suggest some words to them and let them agree or disagree: "Would you describe your pain as 'throbbing'? Would you say your pain is dull or sharp?" Patients should be encouraged to use graphic examples if single words do not seem sufficient. A patient might say, "The pain feels as if someone is shoving a hot, red poker into my back."

Where Is the Pain Located?

Asking the patient to point to the area of pain is useful. If the area can be indicated with one finger, the pain is probably well localized. Patients who have been experiencing severe, prolonged pain may be unable to say where the pain is. Finally, having the patient point to or touch the area where the pain is felt most strongly removes any misunderstanding caused by misuse of descriptive terms. Patients and health professionals often have totally different definitions for certain anatomical locations. For example, a patient who describes a pain as being located in the stomach may mean that the pain is located in the gastric region or, conversely, may think stomach indicates an area as low as the suprapubic region. Pointing with a finger or laying a hand on the area reduces the possibility of miscommunication. Another option is to show the drawings in the pain assessment tool in Appendix A to the patient and have the patient point to the areas where he or she is having pain.

Most cancer patients experiencing pain are experiencing it in more than one region of the body. Patients should always be asked if they are having pain in any other areas. The nurse should not assume that patients will bring up all of their pains spontaneously. Many cancer patients consciously make an effort not to appear like crocks or invalids. If it seems likely that it is important to the patient not to be seen as a complainer, a good start might be a statement such as the following: "Most cancer patients who are having pain actually have discomfort in more than one area. I'm wondering if your (shoulder, back, abdomen, etc.) is the only discomfort you are having or are there other painful areas as well?" If the patient is having more pain, this approach provides an opening for describing the other symptoms. For patients who are not having pain in more than one area, the approach often makes them feel lucky that they are having only one pain.

Does the Pain Radiate Anywhere Else?

Does the pain go somewhere else? Examples are gastric pain that "goes through" to the back and chest pain that "goes down" the arm. This information gives clues as to which dermatomes may be involved and thus provides more insight into which structures are causing the pain. Patients should be asked this question about each pain they are having.

What Are the Temporal Factors?

How long has the pain been present? How does it develop and progress? If a pattern can be detected, interventions started early in the pain course can prevent the full establishment of the pain syndrome. Prevention of severe pain requires less analgesia than treatment does.

Is the pain always present, or does it come and go? The answers to this question provide information essential for determining the potential source of the pain and the types of pain-control measures likely to be effective. Pain that is present most of the time can be treated more easily than pain that occurs for only short periods and then disappears, particularly if the pain is severe.

What Are the Aggravating and Alleviating Factors?

The answers to questions about aggravating and alleviating factors help in diagnosing the potential causes of the pain and give clues to ways to prevent or relieve the pain. Patients are sometimes too involved with their pain, or overwhelmed by it. Consequently, they often cannot see a relationship between certain occurrences and aggravation or relief of the pain. Careful questioning may reveal patterns or relationships that are not obvious to the patient or the patient's family.

What makes the pain worse? Factors that make the pain worse may include eating, not eating, certain activities, sleeping, bowel movements, cold, and so forth. If aggravating factors can be eliminated or modulated, they should be. Twycross gives the example of a patient who always stood to shave every morning, even though this caused severe pain later. An explanation of the relationship between the standing and the later pain—and the arrangement of furniture so the patient could shave sitting down—relieved much of the pain.

What makes the pain better? What activities or cessation of activities appears to make the pain less? Whatever the patient has found to relieve the pain, unless it is harmful in some way, should be incorporated into the pain management plan.

In addition to discovering what movements, positions, home remedies, or other interventions reduce the severity of the patient's pain, the health team also needs to know precisely which medications the patient is taking for pain relief, how frequently the drugs are being taken, what doses are being taken, and how effective the drugs have been. A numerical indication of the intensity of the pain for the patient's records is useful. The patient might be asked, "What is the lowest pain level you usually get after taking your morphine? How soon does your pain start returning?"

Questions about sleep patterns are important. Patients with chronic pain rarely sleep well, and, unless rectified, this can undermine all the other interventions to relieve pain.

The existence of side effects also needs to be specifically asked about. Patients often do not recognize the relationship between their nausea or constipation and the analgesics they are taking.

How Severe Is the Pain?

Questions about the severity of the pain are important, but they are also difficult for a patient with chronic, progressive pain to answer. Patients also get confused about pain severity. They often want to know if the nurse is asking how bad the pain is right at that moment or how bad it was yesterday. A useful response might be, "Let's start with how much pain you are having right this moment." Then, after the patient responds, the nurse could ask, "Would you say the amount of pain you are feeling right now is more or less than you normally experience?" The final questions would be, "When the pain is at its worst, how much pain do you have? What is the least amount of pain you feel?" Whenever possible, a number (on any of the visual analogue scales previously discussed) should be used to describe the severity of the pain. This makes it easier to compare the patient's response to treatment interventions in the future.

It is always a good idea to ask the spouse, adult children, or anyone else who spends a great deal of time with the patient some of the same questions asked the patient. Family members are often much more forthright about the amount of pain that a patient is experiencing. This is particularly useful when the nurse attempting to find out how much pain medication the patient is taking and the amount of pain relief being achieved. Generally, cancer patients tend to downplay how much pain medication they take each 24 hr and exaggerate how well the pain medication works.

GOALS OF TREATMENT

It is essential that all members of the health care team be fully informed about the patient's condition and prognosis. Is the pain due to the cancer, to treatment of the cancer, or to something unrelated to the cancer? Is a cure for the patient's cancer still being sought, or is the patient beyond cure? If cure is no longer possible, what is the estimated life-span of the patient? The answers to these questions determine whether the patient's pain should be approached as acute, chronic benign, or chronic progressive pain.

Patients should be as involved as they want to be with their care. Patients should be kept informed at all times about their prognosis, at a level they are able to cope with (many patients do not want the whole truth). Members of the health team need to understand the patient's view of the situation and know what the patient's expectations and priorities are regarding pain control. For instance, some patients do not think it is possible to relieve severe pain caused by cancer. They may be hoping only to be kept out of agony. Patients with this level of expectation may not report that an analgesic is barely relieving their pain; they do not expect it to.

Other patients think that they will be made completely pain-free. This is not a realistic goal in most situations. These patients need to be educated so that they can develop more realistic expectations about the level of pain control that can be achieved.

For some patients, pain control is not the highest priority. Even patients who are terminally ill may want to continue working as long as possible. In such instances, opioid analgesics, which at least initially cloud the sensorium, may not be wanted. The patient may prefer to tolerate a higher level of pain, to use work as a distraction.

Patients and health care personnel need to work together to clarify the patient's priorities in pain therapy and determine what level of pain relief is realistically possible under those circumstances.

ENSURING PAIN RELIEF

Once a thorough assessment has been completed, it is time to develop a pain treatment plan. A multidisciplinary approach is optimal, allowing input from a variety of specialists, including neurosurgeons, radiotherapists, psychologists, and physical therapists. The health team incorporates this information into a comprehensive treatment plan.

Total pain management in patients in advanced stages of disease should not be undertaken by a solitary professional. Management requires a multidisciplinary group of health professionals working as a cohesive team. The patient and the patient's immediate family should also be considered members of this team.

In those cases in which cancer patients are in severe pain when first seen, a thorough assessment cannot be completed before they have immediate pain relief. This is important for several reasons. First, patients will not be able to cooperate fully when the pain is overwhelming. Second, reducing the pain reassures patients that something can be done to help them. The patient's trust is essential to the future success of any pain management program.

USE OF OPIOIDS IN TERMINALLY ILL CANCER PATIENTS

The significant early advances in the ability to adequately treat pain in terminally ill patients were the result of work in English hospices. Traditionally, opioid analgesics had been used only to manage acute pain. Long-term use had been discouraged because of fear that tolerance, as well as physical and psychological dependence, would develop. Health teams in the hospices rejected traditional approaches to pain management and instead instituted entirely new ways of administering opioid analgesics and other medications to control pain related to cancer. Their success in managing even the most severe pain cases eventually changed the way pain is treated throughout the world.

Major innovations for managing moderate to severe pain were the use of orally administered opioid analgesics and the prevention of pain rather than just the treatment of pain.

Orally Administered Opioid Analgesics

In the United States, before the introduction of these new concepts in pain management, the strongest oral opioid was thought to be Percodan (oxycodone), and outpatients in severe pain were prescribed the ultimate dose: two tablets every 3–4 hr. Occasionally, family members were taught to give Demerol (meperidine) or, less often, morphine injections at home. Otherwise, the use of more potent analgesics was delayed until the patient was thought to be near death and was hospitalized. It was not unusual to hospitalize patients just so that they could be given parenteral opioids. It is not difficult to see why the public (and even professionals) soon began to link the use of parenteral opioids with the end stage of disease.

Prevention of Pain

Perhaps the most profound change was the concept that pain should be prevented, not just treated. That is, pain should be treated *before* it reoccurs. Before this, patients were encouraged—in fact, required—to delay taking additional doses of analgesics until they could not stand the pain any longer. Even when a patient had chronic sustained pain, analgesics were always given on an as needed basis.

The experiences in English hospices showed that this approach was completely wrong. Following it actually led to an increase in pain and opioid requirements. According to Twycross (1978), one of the primary principles of treating chronic cancer pain is, "Thou shall not use the abbreviation p.r.n." Another pioneer in this field, Cicely Saunders, stressed that "constant pain calls for constant control" (Twycross, 1978).

Pain Control in British Hospices

In a retrospective review of 500 patients treated at St. Christopher's Hospice in London, Twycross (1977) described their experience with the use of diamorphine (heroin). More than 80% of the patients received heroin at some time during their stay in the hospice. Nearly 15% of patients taking heroin received it either mostly or exclusively by injection; the remaining 85% took it by mouth in an elixir form. The dose was adjusted to produce analgesia, and the elixir was given regularly in order to produce a continuous pain-free state. Twycross concluded the following:

1. Although, because of increasing debility, parenteral treatment is required during the last 12–48 hr of life in most cases, the majority of patients can be maintained on orally administered heroin before this time.

2. There is no single optimal dose or maximum effective dose of heroin.

3. Use of the prescribed dose of heroin does not, by itself, lead to impairment of mental faculties.

4. Tolerance is not a practical problem.

5. Psychological dependence does not occur.

6. Physical dependence may develop, but it does not appear to prevent the downward adjustment of the dose of heroin when a decrease is considered clinically feasible.

Because of findings such as these, the British concepts of pain treatment arrived on the American shores in the form of Brompton's cocktail.

Brompton's Cocktail

In the early 1970s, tremendous attention was given to a combination of drugs used for controlling pain in terminally ill cancer patients in English hospices. Called Brompton's cocktail, this concoction contained various amounts of heroin, cocaine, a phenothiazine such as Compazine (prochlorperazine), and chloroform water. In some hospices, cocaine was added in the hope that this would counteract some of the sedation caused by the other agents. The following is the original mixture used at St. Christopher's Hospice in London, England:

> Heroin 5 mg (varies)
> Cocaine 10 mg
> Prochlorperazine syrup 5 mg (optional)
> Chloroform water QS to 10 ml
> (volume varies)

It was thought that the ingredients were responsible for the remarkable analgesic effectiveness of Brompton's cocktail. For that reason, it was widely used in the United States to treat severe pain in terminally ill patients. Morphine replaced the heroin, which is illegal in the Untied States. Ultimately, it became obvious, however, that the effectiveness of Brompton's cocktail was not due to its ingredients as much as it was to the manner in which the elixir was administered. The cocktail was given regularly in a dose carefully titrated to the needs of the patient and in a supportive environment in which adequate pain control and maintenance of the patient's quality of life were of paramount importance.

Brompton's cocktail has fallen out of favor because of some of its serious drawbacks. The primary difficulty was that the elixir did not allow sufficient flexibility in tailoring medications to each patient's needs. For instance, the combination of an analgesic with an antiemetic made it necessary to give a patient additional doses of Compazine when all the patient required was additional doses of the opioid. Also, not all patients taking opioids require an antiemetic. Because the phenothiazines can have some serious side effects, it was judged unnecessary to subject all patients to the potential risks unless the patients were actually nauseated. Other ingredients also caused problems. The cocaine caused agitation in a number of patients, and the alcohol added to the depressive effects of the opioids without providing any greater analgesic effect.

Is Heroin Superior to Morphine?

Once it became known that the Brompton's cocktail used in England contained heroin, a movement was begun to legalize the use of heroin in the United States for treatment of pain in terminally ill cancer patients. To determine if heroin was truly superior to morphine, Twycross carried out a controlled crossover trial to compare the effectiveness of these two opioids taken orally. He concluded that when the drugs are given in equianalgesic doses, morphine is a satisfactory substitute for orally administered heroin. His findings agreed with those of earlier researchers. These other studies also showed no detectable differences in the prevalence of side effects (e.g., confusion, nausea, drowsiness). In light of these findings, St. Christopher's Hospice began using orally administered morphine instead of heroin in April 1977.

Yet, the movement in the United States to legalize heroin continues. Some still argue that heroin is more potent per milliliter than morphine and therefore preferable for patients who are being treated with intramuscular or subcutaneous injections of opioids. Dilaudid (hydromorphone), which is readily available in the United States, is nearly identical to heroin in its potency per milliliter (the new concentrated forms are even more potent than equal amounts of heroin). Thus, heroin offers no advantages that are not obtainable through currently available drugs. The problem is not the absence of sufficiently potent drugs. The problem is the improper use of the analgesics already available. Addition of another drug will not solve that problem; it will only add to the confusion.

The Potential Hazards of Meperidine

Meperidine (Demerol) is not the drug of choice for relieving cancer pain. Toxic effects due to its metabolite, normeperidine, are a potential hazard. Normeperidine is a central nervous system stimulant that produces anxiety, tremors, myoclonus, and generalized seizures when it accumulates with repetitive dosing (Kaiko et al., 1983). Patients with renal dysfunction are particularly at risk. Naloxone does not reverse this hyperexcitability; it is an antagonist for the meperidine, not the normeperidine. Because cancer patients are likely to receive repeated doses, they should not be given this analgesic.

CURRENT PRACTICES IN ADMINISTRATION OF ANALGESICS

Although several potent analgesics have been developed, improvement in pain control in cancer patients is primarily due to improvements in the manner of drug administration.

Oral Analgesics

Today, the approach to controlling pain related to cancer starts with a careful assessment of the patient's situation. The next step, when indicated, is prescribing the mildest oral analgesic and noninvasive techniques that will prevent the pain. If the pain is relatively persistent, the analgesics are ordered on a regular, not an as needed, basis, with additional measures or doses to be taken if the pain intermittently flares up. The health team makes certain that the patient is also getting sufficient sleep.

If the pain progresses or recurs after being controlled for a time, the patient's situation is thoroughly reassessed to rule out causes for the pain that are amenable to treatments other than analgesics (e.g., surgery, radiation therapy, antidepressants, antianxiety drugs). If the use of more analgesics is indicated, a more potent opioid analgesic is prescribed to be taken in oral form. Antiemetics, hypnotics, or antianxiety medications may be added to the regimen as the need arises. They are not automatically included in every patient's pain management protocol. Careful assessment and education of the patient continue throughout this process.

For most patients, a pain-free state can be achieved. In the case of morphine, because the therapeutic ratio is not large, the aim is to keep the plasma concentration of morphine within the zone of efficacy but below toxic levels (refer back to Figure 6-2). The dose of opioid is carefully titrated to the point of pain relief by using a regular schedule of oral doses at intervals based on the duration of the clinical effect of the opioid in that patient (for morphine, this is usually 4 hr). The nighttime dose is omitted only when the patient can sleep through the night free of pain. Careful attention to the exact dosage and timing for each patient greatly improves the results achieved. For hospitalized patients, the nurse's input is extremely important because it is the nurse who closely monitors their responses to changes in therapy. Patients who are at home should be instructed to keep a 24-hr diary of their symptoms, activities, food and drug intake, and sleep patterns to help determine the proper dose and best schedule for their analgesics.

Oral doses reach their peak plasma concentrations more slowly and also diminish more slowly than doses given parenterally and thus are safer. The peak drug concentration is higher after parenteral administration. Thus, physicians and nurses should be aware that the plasma concentration may reach a toxic level when a drug is given parenterally, even when an equianalgesic dose is administered. This is rarely a serious problem, however.

During titration of the dose to the level required for good pain relief, changes in the dose can be made at intervals of 24–48 hr and even more frequently if the patient is not experiencing significant relief. While the titration is in progress, further relief can be achieved by using supplemental oral or parenteral morphine when pain control is insufficient.

Table 11-2 shows the usual size of the increments used for titrating a patient's analgesic dose. Note that as the number of milligrams per dose increases, so does the size of the sequential increments.

The maximum effective oral dose of morphine—if one exists—is not known. Recent experience suggests that continuing effectiveness can be obtained with oral doses of 150 mg or more. The limiting factor is the number of pills the patient must swallow, rather than a lack of efficacy above that level. However, most patients have excellent pain relief with 30 mg or less of morphine or an equivalent dose of a morphinelike drug. It is important that the patient understands that oral doses of morphine are as effective as doses given parenterally.

Controlled-release morphine tablets allow longer duration of analgesia than is possible with regular tablets. This is particularly useful during the night. Patients do not have to be awakened to take additional doses. However, nurses must calculate the

TABLE 11-2
Dose Increments for Titration of Analgesic Doses of Morphine

Increment (mg)	Dose Range (mg)
5	2.5–20
10	20–60
20–30	More than 60

equianalgesic dose of morphine for the patient's current drug therapy before starting treatment with controlled-release tablets. First, a total 24-hr daily dose of standard oral morphine is determined. This dose is divided by two (for twice-a-day administration) or three (for three-times-a-day administration) to establish appropriate dosages of controlled-release morphine.

The analgesic drugs commonly used for oral administration and their equianalgesic doses are listed in Table 7-1 in Chapter 7.

Parenteral Opioids

Some patients are unable to take oral analgesics. Reasons include an inability to swallow properly (debility), persistent nausea or vomiting, obstruction of the gastrointestinal tract, and the large number of tablets to be swallowed. In such instances, opioids can be given by a variety of other routes. Drugs currently used parenterally for control of pain are listed in Table 11-3 along with their equianalgesic doses and duration of action compared with morphine.

Opioids can be given parenterally in a variety of ways (Table 11-4). The choice of delivery method depends on the length of time the patient is expected to require intravenous opioids, the amount of opioids required, whether the patient is ambulatory, and the patient's choice.

Intramuscular. The intramuscular route is the least preferred route of administration for drugs for treatment of persistent pain. It is uncomfortable for pa-

tients, especially if they have little muscle mass, as cancer patients often do. Repeated intramuscular injections lead to scarring and unreliable absorption of the medications. If the intramuscular route must be used, the most concentrated opioid solution should be used. For example, a concentrated form of Dilaudid is available that contains 10 mg of Dilaudid per milliliter of solution. Therefore, a dose equal to 15 mg of morphine would require only 0.22 ml of concentrated Dilaudid solution. This would cause much less tissue trauma when given intramuscularly.

Intravenous. Although intravenous administration of morphine has been used in pain management for many years, its application has been limited primarily to hospitalized patients. Venous-access devices (both external and implanted) now provides safe and convenient entry into the vascular system, obviating frequent changes of the site for intravenous injections. Advanced technology has led to the development of many ambulatory infusion systems that provide a regulated flow of analgesic and can be used on an outpatient basis. These innovations have greatly improved the quality of life for many patients and reduced the time spent in the hospital.

Subcutaneous. The development of more concentrated forms of opioids and miniaturized pumps has led to the increased use of subcutaneous infusions as an alternative to intravenous infusions.

Other Routes of Administration

Rectal. Opioids that can be given effectively by the rectal route include Numorphan (oxymorphone) and

Dilaudid (hydromorphone). The rectal route, when acceptable to the patient who cannot take oral analgesics, is preferable to parenteral routes because of fewer complications.

Sublingual. Sublingual forms of morphine and several other analgesics are being tested experimentally. The advantages of this route are obvious. Patients who are unable to swallow tablets would still be able to take analgesics without use of injections or rectal suppositories. Also, the onset of action would be more like the onset after intravenous administration than like the onset after oral administration. Thus, patients who have sudden spasms of pain would be able to take a rapid-onset medication on their own. They would not have to wait for the nurse to prepare an opioid.

Transdermal. Recently, fentanyl has become available in a transdermal patch (Duragesic) that delivers the drug through the skin. Application is simple, and one patch lasts 72 hr. The Duragesic patch is indicated for continuous pain requiring high dosages. Its main disadvantage is that initial evaluation for maximum analgesic effect cannot be made until 24 hr after application; the fentanyl is gradually delivered from the patch and then slowly absorbed through the skin. Patients should be instructed to not expect immediate relief, and additional short-acting analgesics may be required for the first 12–24 hr. Conversion ratios from oral and intravenous opioids are available from the manufacturer of the patch. However, the ratios are conservative, and the patient may need an increased dose. When administration is being changed from the patch to other routes, half the dose of the new opioid should be started within 12–18 hr after removal of the patch. It takes up to 17 hr for the serum levels of fentanyl to fall by 50% after the patch has been removed. The transdermal route allows continuous infusion of high doses of fentanyl without the equipment or invasive procedures required with parenteral routes.

Intraspinal Opioids

Another new method of providing pain relief for cancer patients, one that provides many of the same benefits as PCA, is intraspinal administration of opioids. Use of intraspinal opioids was started in an effort to avoid many of the undesirable central nervous system side effects seen with systemic administration (McQuire, 1987). Opioids administered via the spinal route, either epidurally, intrathecally (subarachnoid), or intraventricularly, produce analgesia directly by their effect on opioid receptors. Minimal amounts of the drug reach supraspinal centers, obviating the central nervous system side effects seen with oral and parenterally administered opioids.

Morphine, levorphanol, hydromorphone, and methadone have all been administered intraspinally. They have also been delivered by repeated boluses vs. continuous infusion and by external vs. subcutaneous catheters and injectable systems. In a review, Benedetti (1987) drew the following conclusions:

1. In about 55–60% of patients with cancer pain, intraspinal opioids will provide good pain relief over a long period.

2. An indwelling subcutaneous catheter with an injection port has advantages over the external epidural catheter, especially in decreasing the prevalence of infection and requiring less frequent replacement.

3. Continuous intraspinal infusion provides better and more uniform pain relief than repeated boluses do.

The most frequently reported side effects of intraspinal opioids include pruritus, nausea and vomiting, urinary retention, somnolence, and respiratory depression. The respiratory depression is usually delayed and can be life threatening. Moderate to severe respiratory depression may occur up to 24 hr after the first administration of intraspinal opioids. Although this has been reported mostly with intrathecal morphine, it also occurs sporadically with

TABLE 11-3
Parenteral Analgesics and Equianalgesic Doses for Moderate to Severe Pain

Agent	Route	Equianalgesic Dose (mg)	Duration Compared with Morphine
Opioid Agonists			
Morphine	IM/IV, etc.	10	Same
Codeine	IM	130	Slightly shorter
Fentanyl (Sublimaze, Innovar)	IM/IV, etc.	0.2	Much shorter
Heroin*	IM	5	Slightly shorter
Levorphanol (Levo-Dromoran)	IM/IV	2	Same
Hydromorphone (Dilaudid)	IM/IV, etc.	5	Slightly shorter
Meperidine (Demerol)	IM/IV, etc.	75	Shorter
Methadone (Dolophine)	IM	10	?
Oxymorphone (Numorphan)	IM	1	Slightly shorter
Mixed Agonist-Antagonists			
Butorphanol (Stadol)	IM	2	Same
Nalbuphine	IM	10	Same
Pentazocine	IM	60	Shorter
Partial Agonists			
Buprenorphine	IM	0.4	Same

* Not legal in the United States

Note: IM = intramuscular, IV = intravenous.

epidural administration. In most patients, slow respiratory rate and apnea will develop. In others, especially older patients, the respiratory rate will remain normal, but tidal volume will decrease severely, and severe hypercarbia and hypoxia will develop if the patient does not receive supplemental oxygen.

The use of intraspinal opioids for the control of pain is still evolving. It is not the universal technique for long-term analgesia. However, when used properly, it provides intense analgesia for many different types of pain. For long-term analgesia, it should be used only when other, simpler forms of pain therapy, such as oral opioids, are no longer effective or the side effects are unbearable.

Summary

Despite improvements in the ability to relieve pain with invasive measures, in some instances, these measures are not successful. For example, specific types of pains, such as neuralgias, spasms, and radiating nerve root pain, do not respond well to opioids, no matter how the drugs are administered. In such instances, other pain management techniques must be used.

In other cases, patients who are receiving doses of opioids sufficient to cloud their sensorium will still complain of inadequate pain control. In these cases, the role of nonphysical factors such as anxiety, repressed anger, and depression should be carefully explored. Careful questioning of patients about their fears and other intense feelings will sometimes re-

TABLE 11-4
Advantages and Disadvantages of Various Methods of Parenteral Drug Administration

Method of Delivery	Drawbacks and Advantages
Intravenous "slow push"	This is a useful method of providing intermittent additional doses of opioids. Because intravenous drugs generally act more quickly, the patient receives more rapid pain relief. The drawback is that the relief does not last as long with IM administration. Also, intermittent "pushes" increase the possibility of phlebitis.
Subcutaneous infusion	This method provides a steady blood level of opioid in patients who do not have a ready venous access. Subcutaneous infusion sets or 27-gauge butterfly needles are inserted into the subcutaneous tissues. Tubing connects the needle to an ambulatory infusion device to provide a continuous delivery of analgesic. Insertion sites can be changed as infrequently as once per week. The chest wall, abdomen, and thigh are frequent sites for infusion.
Continuous intravenous infusion	This technique has been widely accepted in the past decade for treating patients who are terminally ill. More recently, it has been used to treat severe pain in patients who have persistent, steady pain who cannot take sufficient oral doses of opioids. The development of miniature infusion pumps for outpatient ambulatory use has led to more frequent use of this technique in patients who remain mobile.

veal the emotional source of their pain. If depression appears to be a major contributing factor, which is not unusual with prolonged pain, a tricyclic antidepressive can be added to the patient's treatment regimen. Excessive anxiety can often be controlled with the addition of an anxiolytic such as Vistaril. The possibility that the pain is not being controlled because of disease progression or new complications should also be considered.

PROBLEMS RELATED TO PAIN AND ITS MANAGEMENT

Insomnia

Sleep problems almost invariably accompany chronic pain. This lack of adequate rest is a major problem for these patients. Twycross (1985) stresses: "The initial target [of pain-control interventions] should be a pain-free, sleep-full night. . . . To sleep through the night and wake refreshed is a boost to both the doctor's and the patient's morale." When opioids are given for pain relief, the accompanying sedation may solve the problem, but only for awhile. The patient may require additional assistance in obtaining a full night's sleep on a regular basis.

Noninvasive methods should be tried first. Relaxation, applications of heat and cold, and other methods that reduce tension and pain can be effective in improving sleep. If these are not adequate, sedative and hypnotic medications can be added, but care must be taken. Many hypnotics, for instance, lose their effectiveness after a short time. They also can cause abnormal daytime behavior. That is one reason oral antihistamines (e.g., Benadryl [diphenhydramine]) or hydroxyzine (Vistaril) are useful sleeping aids. Also, the total daily dose of a tricyclic antidepressant given at bedtime may be helpful in promoting sleep.

Opioid Side Effects

No matter how carefully the doses are titrated, most patients will experience some adverse side effects from their opioid analgesics, particularly when the drugs are first started. Most of these effects can be overcome.

Nausea and vomiting. Nausea and vomiting are common side effects of taking opioids. Two different sites of action may be involved: the medullary center and the middle ear. The supposed involvement of the inner ear explains the relationship between walking and nausea. The more ambulatory the patient is, the more likely are nausea and vomiting. Therefore, patients should be advised to avoid unnecessary walking during the first days of opioid use.

Antiemetics are often necessary to treat the nausea and vomiting. According to McCaffery (1979), when the initial doses of a phenothiazine antiemetic do not control the nausea, instead of increasing the dose of phenothiazine, an antihistamine antiemetic such as Dramamine could be added. The antihistamine affects a different vomiting mechanism than do the phenothiazines.

After the first 48–72 hr on opioids, the nausea often declines or disappears. Therefore, phenothiazines are often started along with the opioids and then, if possible, discontinued a few days later.

Patients who have persistent nausea with one opioid will not necessarily have similar problems with another opioid. Any patient who is having persistent nausea should be switched to an equianalgesic dose of another type of potent analgesic.

Constipation. Opioids reduce peristalsis in both the small and large intestines, so the stool moves very slowly through the gastrointestinal tract. This allows additional water to be absorbed from the stool, and the stool becomes hard. Constipation is an almost invariable outcome of opioid therapy unless preventive measures are started early.

Mrs. L. was in the advanced stages of breast cancer, with numerous metastatic bone lesions and several pathological fractures. Despite her condition, she refused to take the potent analgesics her physician had ordered for her, denying that she needed them. The nurses thought that she was having severe pain despite her denials, and they asked a pain specialist for help.

During the subsequent assessment, it was discovered that in the past, Mrs. L. had been taking potent opioid analgesics, and fecal impaction had developed. She said that the distress she experienced before and during the removal of the impaction was so great that she could not risk ever getting so severely constipated again. That was why she was refusing potent pain medications.

This case illustrates that distress from constipation can be sufficient to make a patient refrain from taking opioids. Such situations would not occur if patients and their families were properly instructed on how to prevent and treat this miserable side effect.

If possible, the patient should drink plenty of fluids, and keep as active as possible. If the patient is also nauseated, additional activity is contraindicated. If the patient can tolerate them, ingestion of foods high in bran can help by adding bulk. Patients who take bulk-forming laxatives and do not drink enough fluids are at risk of the ingested fiber forming an impaction. These laxatives require good fluid intake.

In most cases, medication is necessary to prevent constipation. Both a stool softener and a mild peristaltic stimulant are needed. Peri-Colace (casanthranol and docusate sodium) has both these effects, and one or two capsules can be given at bedtime. Constipation is one of the last side effects to which patients become tolerant as time passes. Therefore, it is not unusual for high doses of power-ful bowel stimulants to be required to overcome the effects of the high doses of opioids.

Allergy. A true allergic reaction to morphine or other opioids is quite rare, but it does occur. Signs and symptoms are rash, pruritus, and dyspnea or, after injection, an itchy wheal-and-flare response at the site of injection. These can be treated with antihistamines. The opioid should be changed, to an agent with a chemical structure substantially different from the one that induced the allergic reaction.

Tolerance. Tolerance is not the same as addiction. Tolerance occurs in all patients who consistently take opioids for many weeks or months. The earliest indication of developing tolerance is the patient's complaint that the duration of effective analgesia has decreased. If the patient's disease has not progressed, and no new problem is causing additional pain, the most likely explanation is that the patient is becoming tolerant to the opioid. Interestingly, the rate at which tolerance develops depends on the route of administration. Tolerance occurs more slowly with oral opiates and more rapidly with opiates given parenterally. Careful titration of doses slows the development of tolerance considerably. According to some experts, in many cases, no tolerance develops despite several years of opioid therapy.

The treatment for tolerance is to increase the dose or the frequency with which the opioid is administered. Cross-tolerance among opioid analgesics is not usually complete, so sometimes switching from one opioid to another can provide more adequate pain control with less medication. The drugs must be equal in potency. If the new drug is significantly more effective, the starting equianalgesic dose should be slightly lower than that used with the previous medication.

COANALGESICS

Even when used correctly, opioid analgesics do not always relieve cancer pain. In some patients, inadequate relief may indicate the need for nondrug treatment such as radiation. In others, it may indicate the need for a coanalgesic (Table 11-5). Adding nonopioid analgesics to a treatment regimen that includes opioid analgesics can be beneficial, particularly in prolonged pain states. The obvious benefits are that the nonopioids have different side effects and different modes of action.

Tranquilizers

Tranquilizers, especially promethazine (Phenergan), are generally used as potentiators. Table 11-6 indicates the usefulness of various tranquilizers in the treatment of prolonged pain.

Tricyclic Antidepressants

Tricyclic antidepressants are one of the more exciting developments in the treatment of chronic pain. Those commonly used include amitriptyline (Elavil, Endep), doxepin (Sinequan), imipramine (Tofranil), and nortriptyline (Aventyl, Pamelor). The usual recommendation is a total daily dose of 75 mg, although this is adjusted to meet the patient's needs. An effective dose seems to be one that is just enough to cause sedation and dry mouth. Sometimes, an initial dose of 25 or 50 mg at bedtime is increased until the patient reports these symptoms.

Tricyclic antidepressants are usually used to treat endogenous, rather than reactive, depression. Because the depression associated with chronic pain is usually described as reactive, it is thought that the tricyclic antidepressants exert their effect on pain by another mechanism in these patients. The analgesic effects appear to be the result of effects on both the central and the peripheral nervous systems. As discussed in chapter 3, centrally, reuptake of the neurotransmitter serotonin is inhibited, which allows modulation of the pain. This seems to lead to a depersonalization of the pain. Peripherally, the drugs may interfere with the production of pain-producing biochemical substances.

These drugs usually require daily administration for a minimum of 2–3 weeks before their antidepressant effects are noticeable. Patients who have chronic pain, however, may note an analgesic effect in less than 10 days. Patients and family members should be made aware of the lag between the start of therapy and the onset of effects.

Tricyclic antidepressants are also combined with tranquilizers for good effect (e.g., imipramine plus haloperidol [Haldol], a major tranquilizer and an antiemetic). Nortriptyline plus carbamazepine (Tegretol, an anticonvulsant) produced complete pain relief in a group of patients with postherpetic neuralgia.

Tricyclic depressants are sedating. This side effect is usually used to good effect by giving patients their total daily dose at bedtime, early enough so that they do not have continuing drowsiness the next morning.

Muscle Relaxants

Muscle spasm can be precipitated by anxiety or associated with underlying bony metastases. In patients who have muscle spasm, often a tender bone can be palpated, and metastatic bone involvement can be confirmed radiologically. Both diazepam (Valium) and chlorpromazine (Thorazine) have muscle-relaxing properties and are used in the treatment of muscle spasm. Less sedating muscle relaxants can be used in patients who do not want additional sedation. The usefulness of splinting or relief of weight-bearing should not be overlooked in patients with bone metastases.

TABLE 11-5
Coanalgesics for Pain in Cancer

Type of Pain	Coanalgesic
Bone pain	Aspirin, 600 mg every 4 hr or a potent antiinflammatory such as Motrin or Feldene
Raised intracranial pressure	Dexamethasone, 2–4 mg 3–4 times per day; diuretics
Nerve pressure pain	Dexamethasone, 2-4 mg once to twice a day
Superficial dysesthesias	Elavil, 25–100 mg at night
Intermittent stabbing pain	Tegretol (Carbamazepine), 200 mg 2–4 times per day
Gastric distension pain	Maalox Plus or other antacid with simethicone after meals; metoclopramide, 10 mg every 4 hr.
Rectal tenesmoid pain	Chlorpromazine 10–25 mg every 4–8 hours; or rectal belladonna alkaloids 0.2 mg (B&O suppositories)
Muscle spasm pain	Diazepam, 5 mg twice a day
Lymphedema	Diuretics

Source: Adapted from Twycross & Hanks, 1984.

Anticonvulsants

The value of phenytoin (Dilantin) and carbamazepine (Tegretol) in the treatment of neuralgia has been well known for a number of years. As discussed in chapter 3, these drugs stabilize the nociceptor membrane, resulting in a decrease in the pain signal. Less appreciated is the relief these types of drugs can provide for the stabbing pains of postherpetic neuralgia, a relatively common problem in elderly cancer patients. Anticonvulsants are also used to treat the stabbing pain that occasionally occurs with nerve compression due to a neoplasm.

Corticosteroids

Corticosteroids are useful in the treatment of cancer patients in advanced or terminal stages of disease. However, some physicians are still reluctant to use these drugs except for traditional indications.

Corticosteroids can be used in a nonspecific way to improve a patient's mood and appetite, or they may be indicated as specific adjuncts to treatment of a number of cancer pain syndromes (Table 11-7). Their use in pain relief usually involves shrinking the edematous tissue that often surrounds tumors. Tumors often cause pressure on neighboring veins and lymphatic vessels, leading to local or regional edema. The same mechanism underlies the usefulness of corticosteroids in the treatment of increased intracranial pressure. The improvement associated with use of these drugs can last for weeks, or sometimes months, after treatment is started.

Side effects are common with corticosteroids, especially when high doses are used. The most common problems are oral candidiasis (30–35% of patients), edema (20%), and moon face (15–20%). Patients being treated with the most potent form of corticosteroid, dexamethasone, are most likely to experi-

TABLE 11-6
The Usefulness of Tranquilizers in the Treatment of Prolonged Pain

Generic Name	Trade Name	Effective?	Comments
Promethazine	Phenergan	No	Increased sedation.
Chlorpromazine	Thorazine	Perhaps when given on regular schedule	Orthostatic hypotension; when given with narcotic may aggravate respiratory depression.
Promazine	Sparine	Same as with Thorazine	Less than with Thorazine
Hydroxyzine	Atarax Vistaril	Yes	100 mg intramuscularly appears to be equianalgesic to 8 mg of morphine; when combined with morphine, increases potency of morphine by 40%. No increased respiratory depression when combined. Good antiemetic activity without orthostatic hypotension. Not useful when used orally.
Diazepam	Valium	Probably not	Increased sedation is a problem. In some patients, it appears to have some analgesic effect; in others, it increases sensitivity to pain.

ence psychological disturbance and hyperactivity. Peptic ulcers are also seen in a small percentage of patients.

Amphetamines

Amphetamines are powerful stimulants, and the potential for abuse is high. Tolerance to their effects tends to develop rapidly, so they are usually used only in the end stage of disease or for short periods in patients with pain requiring high doses of opioids. Amphetamines have a strong analgesic effect. Most likely they act as a potentiator of morphine or other opioid analgesics. One of the biggest advantages of amphetamines is their ability to offset the sedating effect of opioids. When terminally ill patients re-

quire sudden increases in analgesia during their last days, the addition of an amphetamine allows them to remain alert and pain-free so that family interaction is possible.

GOALS OF PAIN MANAGEMENT

Although the ultimate goal of pain management is always complete freedom from pain, the health team and the patient will be less discouraged if they aim at "graded relief" (Twycross, 1978). Graded goals should include the following.

- Restful sleep. This is an essential first goal. Unless the patient begins to get some restful sleep at night, adequate control of pain is difficult.

- Relief from pain while at rest. Once the patient has had some nights of good sleep, the next goal is to make the patient comfortable at rest. This goal should be achievable in all patients. In some patients, it is achieved fairly rapidly. In others, particularly those who have pain on movement and those whose pain is compounded by extreme anxiety or depression, it may take 3–4 weeks of intensive treatment to achieve satisfactory control. However, in all patients, it should be possible to achieve some improvement within the first 24–48 hr.

- Freedom from pain on movement. This goal is not always attainable. Usually a variety of pain management strategies are required to reduce pain on movement to an acceptable level.

- Erasing the memory of pain. Consistent pain prevention will eventually lead to a lessening of the anxious anticipation and memory of pain. The result is frequently a reduction in the opioid dose required to control the pain.

- An unclouded sensorium. Patients often feel trapped between perpetual pain on the one hand and perpetual somnolence on the other (Mount, 1984). The balance, a state of relative comfort without sedation, requires careful titration of the analgesic dose. This can only be achieved with careful monitoring of the patient's needs and responses to therapy.

OVERWHELMING PAIN

Patients who are experiencing overwhelming pain can be difficult to work with initially because they are so withdrawn (or in a few instances, agitated) and distrusting of the health team's ability to relieve the pain. The key to success with these patients is breaking the cycle of pain-anxiety-insomnia-fatigue-pain. It may take as long as 3–6 weeks to achieve maximum pain relief, because the patient is so exhausted and demoralized. This must be understood by staff members and the patient or they may become demoralized when the pain is still a problem after several days of treatment. Nevertheless, the patient should be promised some early improvement, particularly with regard to rest and comfort at night.

TABLE 11-7
Uses for Corticosteroids in Patients with Terminal Cancer

Nonspecific Uses	Specific Uses	As a Coanalgesic
Improve appetite	Hypercalcemia	Raised intracranial pressure
Enhance mood	Spinal cord compression	Nerve compression
Improve strength	Obstructions by tumors	Head and neck tumors
Reduce fever sweats	Reduction of radiation-induced edema and erythema	Metastatic arthralgias

Source: Adapted from Twycross & Hanks, 1984.

Overwhelming pain should be viewed as an emergency, and adequate time and attention will be required to optimally assist the patient. The first few days are particularly important, because a satisfactory, trusting relationship needs to be established with the patient and the patient's family. The patient's response to early interventions also should be monitored. Treatment usually begins with both a potent analgesic and an antianxiety agent. The doses and types of medications are determined by the physician and are based on what the patient has been taking.

Mount (1984) advises that in cases of excruciating pain, treatments should begin with a higher dose of opioid than is thought to be needed to control the patient's pain. Then small sequential decreases should be made in the dose until analgesia without excessive sedation is achieved (Figure 11-2). Patients who are totally exhausted can be kept heavily sedated for 1–2 days after the start of active interventions to control pain. This allows them the opportunity to receive plenty of rest and reassures them that something is strong enough to control the pain.

Sometimes patients do not want to stop the analgesic they have been taking, even though it has been inadequate, particularly at night. If this is the case, the patient can continue to take the analgesic. The new one is just added to the treatment regimen.

EDUCATION

Persons in the United States are barraged on a daily basis with antidrug information on television and radio and in the newspaper. Consequently, many are tremendously reluctant to take analgesics or mood-altering drugs of any type. The first thing many patients tell the health professional is, "I'm not the type of person to take medicines. Up until recently, I hadn't taken so much as an aspirin in the last 10 years." Inducing these patients to take doses of analgesics, often powerful analgesics, on a regular basis—even when they are not in pain—takes patience and persistence. Patients who are in a great deal of pain are more open to taking their analgesic drug on a regular schedule. Even these patients, however, will try to skip doses once the pain is under control, because they do not like taking medications.

Patients with advanced cancer who are taking regular doses of potent opioids often ask, "Will I always have to take these drugs?" This question includes a number of different concerns: "Does this mean I am going to die soon? Only people who are really close to dying are put on these types of medications, aren't they?" or "Am I going to be dependent on taking drugs all the rest of my life?"

It is useful to compare the need to take regular doses of opioids with the need for regular doses of insulin in patients who have diabetes. The body of a person with diabetes cannot meet its need for insulin, just as the nervous system of a patient with cancer cannot meet its need for high levels of endorphins (the body's own opioid). The nurse should explain that a patient will be able to tell if the need for opioid analgesia has decreased, because the patient will become much more sleepy. At that point, the drug can be stopped or the dose decreased without any problems. Patients with cancer are not addicted to opioids any more than patients with diabetes are addicted to insulin. Both groups both have a chemical deficit that is being treated with replacement therapy.

Patients who have pain relief with regular doses of opioids eventually begin to wonder if the source of the pain has disappeared and they are taking unnecessary or too much pain medication. At this point, the nurse should reexplain the rationale for not skipping doses or returning to an as needed schedule, and tell the patient that if the dose of opioid were too high, the patient would be very sedated. However, the patient will probably still try skipping doses. Depending on the type of opioid analgesic

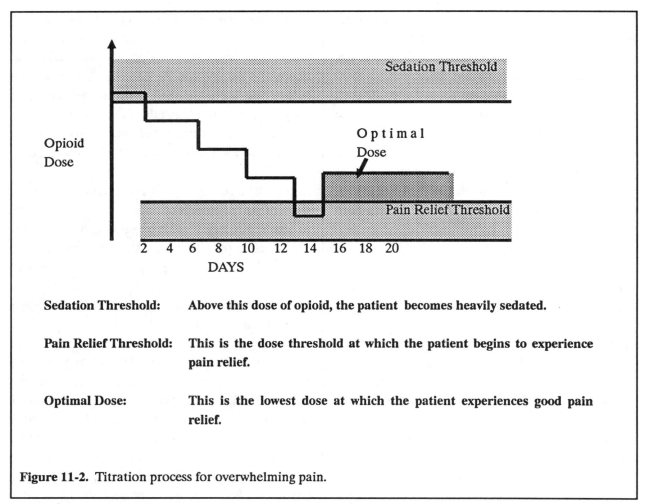

Figure 11-2. Titration process for overwhelming pain.

being taken, the pain may not return for several days. When the pain does reappear, it is usually sufficient proof to the patient that the source of pain is still present. Occasionally the pain will become uncontrolled if a sufficient number of doses have been skipped, particularly if the patient is taking a long-acting pain medication such as methadone. More frequent doses of the analgesic may be required for a period to get the patient comfortable again.

Another important topic for education is the prevention of constipation. This is particularly true for outpatients who may think that they can control the situation with a little extra fiber or fluid. The nurse should explain that prevention of constipation is just as important as prevention of pain.

The preventive approach also must be stressed with regard to the control of nausea. Foremost, at the start of treatment with opioids, the patient should be given a prescription for an antiemetic, both oral and rectal forms, to be used as needed for nausea. Outpatients should be advised to have both prescriptions (analgesic and antiemetic) filled at the same time. Otherwise the time between the onset of nausea and the taking of the antiemetic may be prolonged while the patient waits for the antiemetic to be brought home. Patients tend to wait until the nausea has progressed to vomiting before they take the antiemetic. They should be informed that the nausea usually passes after several days and that movement can make it worse. They should be encouraged to take the antiemetic sooner rather than later during the first few days and to avoid unnecessary movement.

AHCPR GUIDELINES

The AHCPR is expected to publish clinical practice guidelines for the management of cancer pain in 1994. For definition and explanation of the role of clinical practice guidelines, see chapter 8.

SUMMARY

The key concepts stressed in this chapter include the following:

1. Use a preventive approach to pain. Medication should be administered before pain recurs or before it increases. Use regular doses if the source of pain is consistent.

2. Start with nonopioid analgesics whenever possible for mild to moderate pain. Use antiinflammatories even in severe pain when production of prostaglandins is a major component in the painful process.

3. Do not overlook the efficacy of noninvasive pain-relief methods, even when potent analgesics are being administered. These methods can greatly enhance the effectiveness of the analgesics.

4. Oral administration of analgesics is always preferable to parenteral administration for regular relief of pain. Parenteral administration can be used for flare-ups of pain or as pretreatment for painful procedures, times when faster onset of action is desirable.

5. During the initial stages of getting a patient's moderate or severe pain under control, reassure the patient that the pain will soon be better controlled. Remind the patient of improvement that has been achieved, and explain the graded, long-term approach to pain management.

6. Never delay use of opioids because of a fear of tolerance, psychological addiction, or respiratory depression.

7. When the patient must be changed from parenteral to oral analgesics, oral to parenteral drugs, or from one analgesic to another, always be careful that equianalgesic doses are administered. Watch closely for signs that the dose of the new medication is excessive or inadequate. If necessary, contact the physician immediately to readjust the dose.

8. Watch closely for an increased need for analgesia. This may be due to an increase in the amount of pain produced by the disease, increasing tolerance to the opioid analgesic, or another cause (e.g., constipation) that can be treated by other methods. When the increased pain is not due to a cause that can be relieved by other interventions, the patient's analgesics should be increased, either by increasing the dose or decreasing the intervals between doses.

9. As opioids are always constipating, use a vigorous approach to prevent constipation.

10. If a patient continues to be oversedated, consider discontinuing antiemetics, potentiators, or other drugs that may be contributing to the sedative side effects of the opioids. (These drugs should be stopped only if their primary effect is thought to be no longer necessary.)

11. Contact the physician if the patient does not respond as expected to changes in pain management. Do not wait for rounds if the patient is in moderate or severe pain.

12. Provide continuous support and education to the patient and the patient's family. Discuss the goals of pain management. Make the patient and the family active participants

in the plan. Explain how harmful unrelieved pain can be to the patient's condition. Explain differences between tolerance and addiction. Explain the need to prevent, not just treat, pain. Teaching and support are critical to the success of interventions for pain management.

EXAM QUESTIONS

Chapter 11

Questions 81-90

81. What percentage of cancer patients with advanced stages of disease experience pain?

    a. 95–100
    b. 60–90
    c. 30–50
    d. 15–25

82. What pain syndrome is associated with the use of vinca alkaloids in the treatment of cancer?

    a. Pseudorheumatism
    b. Trigeminal neuralgia
    c. Migraine headaches
    d. Peripheral neuropathy

83. How are patients with severe chronic pain likely to react when asked what their pain feels like?

    a. They will have vivid descriptions of their pain.
    b. They often have difficulty describing their pain.
    c. They usually get hostile when asked this question.
    d. They usually describe their pain as "throbbing."

84. Which of the following descriptions about time to peak plasma concentration and duration of orally vs. parenterally administered morphine is correct? Oral doses reach peak levels:

    a. More slowly but diminish more quickly.
    b. More quickly but diminish more slowly.
    c. More slowly and diminish more slowly.
    d. More quickly and diminish more quickly.

85. Which of the following tranquilizers is an effective coanalgesic for the treatment of prolonged pain?

    a. Xanax
    b. Valium
    c. Sparine
    d. Vistaril

86. What side effect has been associated with the use of intraspinal opioids?

    a. Kidney failure
    b. Respiratory depression
    c. Liver damage
    d. Cardiac arrest

87. What is the earliest indication that tolerance is developing to an opioid?

    a. The patient is less relaxed than previously.
    b. The amount of analgesia provided has increased.
    c. The analgesic no longer makes the patient drowsy.
    d. The duration of analgesia has decreased.

88. Which of the following is a major innovation in the administration of analgesics for management of moderate to severe pain?

    a. Treating pain 1 hr after its onset
    b. Making patients responsible for the timing of administration
    c. Allowing treatment when the pain begins
    d. Treating pain before it begins

89. What type of coanalgesic is especially useful in the treatment of pain associated with bony metastases?

    a. Anticonvulsants
    b. Corticosteroids
    c. Tranquilizers
    d. Muscle relaxants

90. What type of coanalgesic reduces pain by shrinking the edematous tissue that often surrounds tumors?

    a. Anticonvulsants
    b. Corticosteroids
    c. Tranquilizers
    d. Muscle relaxants

CHAPTER 12

CHRONIC BENIGN PAIN

CHAPTER OBJECTIVE

After studying this chapter, the reader will be able to describe types of chronic pain disorders and the problems related to these disorders.

LEARNING OBJECTIVES

After studying this chapter, the reader will be able to

1. Specify the most common problem, other than the pain itself, of patients with chronic pain syndrome.

2. Specify the chronic benign pain disorder caused by violent deformation of nerves by high-velocity missiles.

3. Select the type of chronic benign pain disorder that has no apparent physical signs in 60–78% of cases.

4. Specify when health care professionals should become concerned about physical dependence in patients taking daily doses of opioids.

5. Specify the term used for family members of patients with chronic benign pain who harm the patients' rehabilitation by continued expressions of sympathy and acts of kindness.

INTRODUCTION

Chronic pain is defined as pain that persists a month beyond the usual course of an acute disease or a reasonable time for an injury to heal. Although many clinicians and researchers use 6 months as an arbitrary cut-off point, some pain specialists think this is inappropriate because a number of acute diseases or injuries resolve or heal in 2, 3, or 4 weeks. In such situations, pain present 4 weeks after a cure should have been achieved must be considered chronic. This has important clinical implications. The earlier such chronic pain syndromes are effectively treated, the better are the chances of cure.

The term benign is frequently attached to the term chronic. As mentioned in chapter 1, the term benign should not be interpreted to mean that no physical abnormality is present. In most patients, a source of chronic pain has been determined. What is not known is how to eliminate the pain. Also, as pointed out in this chapter, benign pain is far from benign. It seriously impairs the patient's physical and mental health and often results in huge bills for unnecessary diagnostic procedures and ineffective treatments.

Nearly 13 of every 100 Americans has some degree of chronic pain. Chronic pain is a serious medical problem. It not only results in lost productivity but also is related to a great deal of drug abuse. Estimates in 1983 suggested that approximately 90 million Americans had chronic pain. Of these, some 60 million were partially or totally disabled for periods ranging from a few days (e.g., for recurrent headaches) to weeks, months, and years (e.g., lower back pain), and some were permanently disabled (e.g., arthritis, lower back pain, cancer pain). This caused a loss of some 700 million workdays. This loss of work productivity, together with health care costs and payments for compensation, litigation, and quackery, totaled nearly $70 billion (Table 12-1). By 1980, more than 800 pain treatment centers had been set up in the United States to treat patients whose lives were being destroyed by pain.

DISORDERS THAT CAUSE CHRONIC BENIGN PAIN

Neuralgias

Several pain syndromes associated with peripheral nerve damage are generally categorized as neuralgia. The clinical features are similar to those of phantom limb pain and causalgia. Neuralgias are characterized by severe, unremitting pain that is difficult to treat by surgical or other traditional methods. The causes include viral infections of nerves, nerve degeneration associated with diabetes, poor circulation in the limbs, vitamin deficiencies, and ingestion of poisonous substances such as arsenic. Almost any infection or disease that produces damage to peripheral nerves, particularly the large nerve fibers, can cause neuralgic pain.

TABLE 12-1
Estimated Prevalence and Cost of Chronic Pain in the United States

Type of Pain	Prevalence, in Millions	Disability, in Millions Partial	Disability, in Millions Total	Total Cost, in Billions ($)
Back pain	23	10	3	23
Painful arthritis	21	6	2	17
Other musculoskeletal	6	4	0.5	2
Severe recurrent headaches				
Migraine	16	16		136
Other	20	20		

Source: Bonica, 1987.

Postherpetic neuralgia is a sequela of infection by the herpesvirus (varicella-zoster virus) that causes chickenpox. Flare-ups of latent virus produce inflammation of one or more sensory nerves. The inflammation, which is painful, is associated with eruptions (or shingles) at the skin at the termination of the nerve. The prevalence of this type of neuralgia is increased in patients with malignant tumors or acquired immune deficiency syndrome, particularly in those patients more than 50 years old. Three types of pain generally occur: continuous burning pain, painful dysesthesias, and intermittent shocklike pain.

The herpetic attack is itself painful, but the pain usually subsides. In a few persons, usually elderly, the pain persists and may even grow more intense after the skin lesions heal. The affected areas of the skin are not only susceptible to spontaneous pain (in the absence of stimulation) but also extremely hyperesthetic, so that the pain is aggravated by any cutaneous stimuli applied to them. Even the friction of clothing may be irritating, and skin contact is avoided as much as possible. The pain may also be intensified by noise in the immediate vicinity or by emotional stress. This condition can last for many months, or even years, and is extremely resistant to most forms of therapy. Some evidence indicates that treatment with corticosteroids during the early stage of herpes zoster (shingles) may prevent or modulate postherpetic neuralgia. Anticonvulsants such as Tegretol (carbamazepine) have also been used, with limited success.

Causalgia

Causalgia is a severe, burning pain characteristically associated with rapid, violent deformation of nerves by high-velocity missiles such as bullets. It is estimated to occur in 2–5% of cases of peripheral nerve injury and is typically seen in young men who have been wounded in military combat. Causalgia persists more than 6 months after injury in 85% of cases and then begins to disappear spontaneously. Nevertheless, 1 year after injury, about 25% of patients still complain of pain.

Causalgia has many of the features of phantom limb pain as well as other unusual characteristics. Its dominant feature is the unrelenting intensity of the pain. Patients have described it as being like a blaze of fire and as if someone were pouring boiling water on top of the foot and holding a lighted cigarette lighter under the big toe (Melzack & Wall, 1983).

The sympathetic nervous system appears to play a particularly important role in causalgia. The affected limb usually shows a variety of signs and symptoms that indicate abnormal sympathetic activity. For example, if the arm is involved, the hand is cold, often drips sweat, and is discolored (presumably due to vascular changes), and even the fingernails become brittle and shiny.

Causalgia, like phantom limb pain, is determined by several factors: sensory inputs from the somatic as well as the auditory and visual systems, activity in the sympathetic nervous system, and cognitive activities such as emotional disturbance. No single factor can be considered the sole cause.

Injection of a local anesthetic into the sympathetic ganglia may dramatically abolish the pain and the abnormal sympathetic signs and symptoms for long periods, sometimes permanently. Sympathectomy, moreover, produces permanent relief.

Lower Back Pain

Lower back pain is one of the most common types of pain, yet it is poorly understood. It shows the complexity of interactions among different contributing factors and the need for multiple approaches in treatment.

The only definite causes of lower back pain are herniation of disks and arthritis of vertebral joints. However, patients with lower back pain do not always have these abnormalities.

Up to 60–78% of patients with lower back pain have no apparent physical cause of pain. That is, radiographs and thorough orthopedic examination show no evidence of disk disease, arthritis, or any other condition that can be considered the cause of the pain.

Even in cases with clear-cut physical and neurological signs of disk herniation (the disk pushes out of its space and presses against nerve roots), surgery provides complete relief of back pain and related sciatic pain in only about 60% of cases (range, 50–95%). Removal of a disk is most likely to be effective in patients with clear evidence of compression of one or more nerve roots.

Many promising therapies for lower back pain have turned out to be less exciting than the original expectation. Injection of papain, an enzyme, to dissolve the disk seemed to be a major advance, but studies showed that it is no more effective than an injection of an inert liquid. Fusion of several vertebrae to provide structural support to unstable vertebrae in patients with lower back pain who have evidence of a herniated lumbar disk was another treatment. However, research showed that fusion is not beneficial and may even be harmful (Melzack & Wall, 1983).

Thus, even when physical causes are clearly present, lower back pain remains a problem after surgery for many patients. In addition to these are the high proportion of patients who have no obvious physical cause.

Lower back pain usually has a particularly unpleasant quality. It is deep, aching, and burning and sometimes immobilizes the patient, who becomes terrified of moving and triggering a severe bout of pain. Often the pain radiates down the leg. This is called sciatic pain because it follows the innervation pattern of the sciatic nerve. For patients with minor physical signs such as curvature of the spine or the normal disk disease that occurs with aging, surgery is rarely effective at relieving the pain. Some of these patients, in a desperate search for relief, prevail on surgeons to carry out successive operations.

A variety of forms of physical therapy may help lower back pain. The most effective is a regimen of special exercises that develop the back muscles. Transcutaneous electrical nerve stimulation, ice massage, and acupuncture may be of some help to some patients. In others, injections of trigger points may be effective.

In many cases of lower back pain, the major culprit may be abnormal activity in nerve-root fibers caused by minor changes in the surrounding vertebrae and tissues. The nerve roots may be affected by compression caused by degenerated disk material (which commonly occurs during normal aging), interference with the blood supply, stress on ligaments and joints that surround the nerve, and so forth. These minor irritations can be cumulative and eventually produce signs and symptoms of lower back sprain. This can be the beginning of a vicious cycle leading to a chronic pain syndrome.

Because of the persistence of lower back pain despite orthopedic surgery, neurosurgery, and countless drugs (most fail to work and some, such as tranquilizers, actually increase depression), psychological therapy has become an important new approach to the problem. Tricyclic antidepressants are sometimes remarkably effective in relieving both the pain and the patient's depression. Effective kinds of therapy include behavior modification, progressive relaxation, hypnosis, and biofeedback to help learn muscle relaxation. All of these help some patients, but no one technique is more effective than the others. What is superior is the use of several treatment techniques at the same time. One clinic found that patients with several different pain syndromes, but mostly lower back pain, were helped by a combination of techniques. About 80% of patients had marked to moderate improvement after treatment, and 50% claimed they still had improvement 3–6 months later. Interestingly, most patients reported that the pain was unchanged, but they were able to work, live with their pain, and lead more normal lives.

WHEN THE PAIN DOES NOT GO AWAY

Acute pain normally begins to disappear within days or weeks of injury as healing becomes complete. Health professionals should become concerned when a patient continues to need opioid analgesics on a daily basis for more than a month after the onset of pain, no matter what the source of the pain. The basis for this concern is that the patient will become physically dependent on an opioid analgesic. When dependency occurs, the pain actually increases in intensity if the patient does not take the medication several times a day.

Secondary Gains

Another concern is that outcomes of the pain may reinforce the patient's pain behavior, for so-called secondary gains. This may or may not be true. McCaffery (1979) gives the following example:

> The patient may use pain as a reason to rest. Resting at work may enable him to avoid a task he does not like, such as inventorying supplies. He is using his pain for secondary gains. However, it is also possible that in spite of disliking the inventory, the reason the patient rests is to relieve the pain, not to avoid the inventory. In this instance pain is not being used for secondary gain purposes. . . . The fact that the patient uses his pain to his advantage does not mean that the pain is of any lesser intensity than the patient reports.

It is possible to derive secondary benefits from pain, even when the pain is very real. This usually does not occur at a conscious level. However, nearly everyone has at some point in life used pain as an excuse to avoid some unwanted activity or event. Therefore, a patient's occasional use of a pain or an ache for a secondary gain does not warrant the health team becoming suspicious about the reality of the patient's pain.

Acute Pain That Is Not Improving

What steps should be taken when the patient's pain seems to be persisting for an indefinite period? The following approaches should be instituted by the health team after an assessment of the patient's condition and situation.

1. The patient should be instructed to take the least potent analgesic that takes the edge off the pain. The patient should also use one or more noninvasive pain-relief measures whenever possible (e.g., TENS, applications of heat or cold, massage). This approach has two advantages: the chance of physical dependence is lessened, and it is much easier to get the patient to eventually eliminate opioid analgesics.

2. The patient should be instructed to take the analgesic on a regular schedule, not as needed for pain. The drug should be taken according to the clock, not according to the severity of the pain. With this approach, the patient does not experience peaks and valleys of pain, because the pain is not allowed to get really bad before another dose of pain medication is taken. Many patients resist taking analgesics before the pain returns, but careful explanation of the benefits of regular doses usually convinces them to give it a try. Also, because the severity of the pain does not determine whether an analgesic is taken, the patient does not need to monitor the pain to decide when it is okay to take another dose.

3. The patient should be encouraged to resume as much activity as possible (see "Activity pacing" in section on pain treatment programs). This helps keep the patient mobile and distracted from the pain and reduces any reinforcement that may be occurring because the patient is able to avoid work, school, and so forth.

CHRONIC PAIN SYNDROME

Unless a great deal of care is taken, chronic pain syndrome is likely to develop in patients who consistently experience pain for 6 months or more. This syndrome is characterized by a number of predictable physical, mental, familial, and social problems (see chapter 11, Figure 11-1.)

Probably the most common complaint of patients with pain is disturbed sleep. Patients say that since the pain started they have had trouble falling asleep because they cannot get comfortable. Then, when they finally find a marginally comfortable position and try to relax, the lack of distracting activities allows the pain to become the focus of their attention, further postponing sleep. Finally, when they do fall asleep, normal movements during the night cause increased pain that awakens them.

Even those few who are able to sleep well report that they feel exhausted all the time. Feelings of irritability and inability to cope are common. Those taking opioids also intermittently have side effects from the drugs, such as nausea, constipation, sedation.

Chronic pain also leads patients to curtail their normal physical activities for fear that the activities will exacerbate their symptoms. As a result, they lose muscle tone and flexibility and start to feel and act as if they were invalids.

Patients with a chronic pain syndrome become socially isolated. Their tendency to talk incessantly about their pain makes others avoid them. In addition, they are often too tired, irritable, and obsessed with their pain to be sociable.

The outcome of all these changes is usually depression and a slow decline into invalidism.

EFFECT OF CHRONIC PAIN ON THE PATIENT'S FAMILY

The effects of persistent pain are every bit as grim for the members of the patient's family as for the patient. It is distressing for family members to see someone they love in pain. Their natural impulse is to try to help in every way they can. They show their concern in many ways: encouraging the patient to rest, bringing the heating pad, or calling the doctor when the pain is especially bad. The outcome is growing frustration when the pain goes on and on with no change for the better in sight.

Furthermore, as time goes by without any relief or answers in sight, the patient becomes more and more cranky and difficult to live with. Suppressed anger and resulting guilt become more intense, interfering with family communications.

Sternbach (1987) also notes that under these circumstances, family members begin to "play games" with each other without consciously realizing what is taking place. Despite the sincerity of their feelings and good intentions, they start trying to manipulate one another in order to get a payoff.

The Tyrant

Pain patients can become a kind of tyrant at home. They get their way with the aid of a powerful weapon: pain. For example, the pain can help the patient to get out of many responsibilities:

Pain patient: "It's not that I don't want to (put out the trash, have sex, go to work). I just can't."

Spouse: "That's all right, dear. I understand."

The pain serves as an honorable excuse. Anyone who insists that the patient live up to the patient's responsibilities is made to appear unfeeling and cruel. It is rarely discussed that the pain itself is not a disability, and that the word "can't" is inaccurate and really means "don't want to."

In addition to getting out of things they would rather not do, tyrants use behaviors such as grimaces, moans, and other indications of severe pain to get others to do things that the tyrants could easily do. In response to the expressions of pain, the concerned family member offers to bring the pills or heating pads or take the patient to the doctor, things the patient could actually do with little or no assistance. Such behaviors extract a tremendous toll:

- They reinforce the patient's sick role. The patient surrenders normal responsibilities and continues having others do what he or she can and should do.

- They put an added burden on the spouse or other family members, who must act as a parent to the childish patient while having no one to reciprocate by providing even normal attention.

Tyrannical behavior is also used against the children in a family. Without actually resorting to discipline, the patient can keep the children under control by overtly expressing pain and producing guilt feelings in them. Thus, these patients tyrannize their homes by avoiding responsibilities, controlling family members' behavior, and deriving the secondary gains of lying around while others do their work for them.

Tender, loving care is appropriate and necessary in the acute pain situation. As the duration of the pain stretches out, with the pain becoming more chronic than acute, patients and their families must be encouraged to resume their normal patterns of activity and ways of dealing with one another.

It must be stressed to family members that it is not their fault that the patient is in pain; they should not feel guilty. They must insist on maintaining their own independent lives. This does not mean, of course, that the patient should be ignored. Normal attention and support should be given, but family members simply should not react to or reinforce the patient's expressions of pain.

Family Sabotage

It is hard for family members to realize that their acts of kindness and expressions of sympathy are actually harmful to the patient with chronic benign pain. The patient must learn how to overcome the pain in order to lead a more normal and satisfying life. Continued expressions of sympathy and doing things for these patients that the patients can for themselves have adverse effects:

- The patient is reminded of the pain, so that it is magnified in his or her awareness.

- The patient is kept from functioning normally and so is kept in a disabled state, unable to do the things he or she would normally be able to do despite pain.

Sternbach (1987) related a story told to him by an ex–Green Beret who was severely injured by a mortar round and had chronic pain:

When I was first hurt, I used to get all this sympathy and pity, you know? The nurses and volunteers, how they'd look at you, you could see what they were thinking. "Oh this poor man. What a shame!" Man, I used to eat it up. I really enjoyed feeling sorry for myself, saying, "Yeah, I've really been shafted."

He received similar expressions of sympathy from friends and family when he went home. They gave me all this tea-and-sympathy crap, and I actually had to tell them to knock it off. That stuff's okay when you're first hurt and feeling sorry for yourself. But after, when you're trying to pull yourself together and adjust and rehabilitate, it's just sabotage.

Family members often must be counseled and educated so that they do not inadvertently sabotage the patient's attempts at rehabilitation. For some family members, however, being in control provides a payoff: it keeps the patient helpless and dependent on them. They actively (but probably not consciously) promote the patient's disability by discouraging efforts at rehabilitation. For instance, when the patient indicates that he or she wants to resume activity, they discourage the effort, warning the patient of all the problems such activity might start. Among pain specialists, a family member who exhibits this type of behavior is referred to as an *enabler* or a *reinforcer* of the patient's excessive disability. Rather than encouraging the patient to participate in the rehabilitation program and to resume a normal life, the spouse or other family member tries to undermine the process by questioning the wisdom of any new exercises or activities prescribed: "Isn't that too much? It will just make the pain a lot worse and may even cause some damage."

This type of communication tends to reinforce the patient's fears and self-doubts and makes the patient overly dependent on the reinforcer, which is just what the reinforcer wants:

> And that of course is the real reason why the relation behaves this way. It is not normal caring or kindness or concern, but has the payoff of giving the relation power and control over the patient in a skewed family relationship. When there is a consistent and repeated pattern of reinforcing disabled behavior and undermining progress, the "concern" is really sabotage. (Sternbach, 1987)

Sometimes, family members become socially isolated along with the patient. Frequently, the family's insurance and savings are depleted by desperate attempts to find a cure for the patient's pain. Everyone becomes increasingly angry and bitter as the months and years go by.

Healthy Coping Strategies for Families

Sternbach (1987) provides family members with useful advice on how they should respond to the patient whose pain is persisting beyond the normal healing time. When it is obvious that the pain is here to stay (certainly after 6 months or so), it is time for a discussion between the members of the patient's family and the health team. Important issues to be clarified at these discussions include the following:

- What is it safe for the patient to do? Can the pain safely be ignored and activities resumed? Families should get specific information. Is there danger of further injury if normal activities are resumed? Can the patient's comfort level be safely used as a guide to the gradual increasing of the patient's activities?

- The family needs to make a plan for getting things back to normal. This obviously cannot be done all at once. If the patient has been essentially out of commission for 6 months or more, a reasonable time schedule needs to be worked out for the patient to gradually resume normal responsibilities.

The overall attitude of the family toward a member with chronic benign pain should be one of patient, hopeful expectation of progress. The family should praise progress and give compliments for each small improvement. They should also ignore all the usual pain behaviors—grunts, moans, sighs, limping, or grasping a painful region—for the patient's own good. The patient must begin acting normal again and give up the sick role and all the characteristics of invalid behavior.

The family should not nag the patient. Sick and disabled behavior must be ignored, not scolded. A parent-child role must be avoided. If the patient is unable to make any notable progress on his or her own, the advice and assistance of a pain treatment center may be required.

PAIN TREATMENT CENTERS

Fortunately, pain treatment centers can help patients with chronic pain syndrome regain a more normal life. The expertise of a team of medical, nursing, and behavioral specialists is usually required. Chronic pain syndrome can be treated on either an inpatient or an outpatient basis.

The first step taken in these centers is to determine if any additional diagnostic or therapeutic strategies might further define or eliminate the source of a patient's pain. If these studies show that the pain cannot be eliminated at that time, the patient is started on a program to teach him or her how to live with the pain.

Many patients are physically dependent on numerous medications when they start these programs. The drugs were prescribed and taken with the best of intentions: to relieve the patient's pain. By the time these patients are recognized as drug abusers, they often have severe physical and psychological problems caused by the medications. Frequent falls, severe memory lapses, falling asleep frequently during the day, and even hallucinations are all signs that a person taking potent opioids on a prolonged basis may be physically dependent on the drugs. Usually the patient needs help to stop taking the harmful medications.

Common Treatment Strategies

Common treatment strategies in pain treatment centers include multiple approaches, physical conditioning, detoxification, goal setting, and activity pacing.

Multiple approaches. A variety psychological techniques are used to enhance the patient's ability to cope constructively with the stress of chronic pain. Patients must unlearn maladaptive or ineffective behaviors that intensify their problems and replace the old behaviors with new, more adaptive ones.

Multiple noninvasive pain-relief techniques are also used: biofeedback, TENS, relaxation, applications of heat and cold, and other methods mentioned in the chapter on methods for controlling pain. The use of analgesics, except occasional use of mild analgesics, is discouraged. Even nonopioid analgesics can lead to increased rebound pain if used consistently over a period of time.

Physical conditioning. An important element in many programs is helping patients overcome their physical disabilities. Most patients are more disabled than necessary because of depression and other factors that encourage inactivity. Their deconditioned, frequently overweight, bodies are more vulnerable to injury (e.g., strains and sprains). Thus, one of the first steps is to start the patient on a conditioning regimen.

Strengthening of specific muscle groups is also an important component of treatment. For example, patients with chronic lower back pain are given exercises to strengthen the abdominal muscles.

Detoxification. Patients often enter these programs dependent on a variety of analgesics, antidepressants, hypnotics, and other powerful medications. One goal is to carefully wean patients off their addictive drugs. Carefully decreasing the doses of drugs avoids the distressing side effects of drug withdrawal.

Some inpatients may be put on a regular schedule of analgesics (referred to as a time-contingency schedule as opposed to a pain-contingency schedule). Every 6 hr is the most common administration interval. The purpose of using a regular schedule is to provide a continuous level of analgesia or to detoxify the patient. With detoxification, the patient is put on a regular schedule of gradually decreasing doses. These patients are carefully selected and are closely observed throughout the process. Sometimes detoxification is necessary to improve a patient's level of consciousness so that a diagnosis can be made. For others, detoxification along with behavioral modification may result in a decrease in pain-related behaviors and a decrease in their requirement for analgesics. Other patients can be switched to drugs with fewer side effects, enabling them to function better.

Goal setting. Patients are assisted in setting realistic goals for their lives and in deciding on specific steps for achieving those goals. Patients with chronic pain tend to just exist, waiting for the day their pain disappears. The aim of the program is help them accept the fact that pain will continue to be a part of their lives for the foreseeable future.

Activity pacing. Patients with chronic pain develop a habit of sitting or lying for extended periods because being active causes them increased pain. Then they become disgusted with themselves and attempt to do too much. The result is a great deal of pain and several days of bed rest. This cycle is repeated again and again. With activity pacing, patients monitor their pain while doing an activity or task. When the pain begins to increase, they stop and lie down to rest for 15 min. During that time, they do relaxation exercises. Before restarting the task or activity, they do a few exercises. With this regimen, many patients are able to improve their endurance considerably.

The Importance of Patients' Attitudes

As with any complex treatment for a complex problem, not all patients are candidates for treatment in pain clinics. Even among those who are, some patients attending these programs will not achieve the desired results. Patients and families can get from a program only what they put into it. Even at best, most patients are still going to experience pain after completing the program. The goal of these programs, and the techniques they teach, is to help patients cope better with pain. Coping better can make a tremendous difference in the quality of the patients' lives.

Sternbach (1987) has identified certain traits that characterize patients who are ultimately able to master their pain problems. Patients who have trouble overcoming their problems usually have misconceptions about the meaning of their pain or have attitudes that interfere with their overcoming it. Some attitudes are basic to learning to live successfully with chronic pain.

Realistic acceptance that the pain cannot be cured. Once the patient has had thorough work-ups by several competent specialists and has been told that the pain cannot be eliminated, the patient must accept the fact. "Doctor shopping" in search of an elusive cure cannot continue indefinitely if the patient is to get on with life. Some conditions such as arthritis, degenerative diseases of the spine, peripheral nerve damage, and thalamic pain associated with a stroke will continue causing the patient pain.

Sternbach provides the example of Sam, a 46-year-old Oklahoman who had already had three operations on his back by the time he was seen in the pain clinic. For 20 years, Sam had been operating bulldozers and tractors during the week, and on weekends, he was a contestant in bronco and steer riding. His spine had undergone severe trauma throughout these years.

> Sam apologizes for standing, but says his back hurts too much to sit. He is 6 feet tall, about 180 pounds, and despite much forced inactivity for the past year, he is hard mus-

cled and trim as a young athlete. He briefly describes his accident, the surgeries (laminectomies and spinal fusions) and tells how he has refused all analgesics despite pain so severe he could barely drive his pickup truck to our clinic.

Sam limps slowly back and forth in my office as he comes to the point of his visit. "When I went back to the doc that operated on me, he said that there was nothing more that he could do and I'd have to learn to live with the pain." Sam's jaw muscles twitch as he blurts out angrily, "Now that's a helluva thing for a doctor to say! I think it's a stupid thing to say. I'm going to get rid of this pain!"

Sternbach asked what Sam would do if the clinic couldn't take the pain away. Sam replied, "Then I'll find someone who will." This patient's attitude is not promising. He will probably not respond to the services offered in the pain clinic. If he persists in trying to find a cure instead of learning to live with his pain, he will probably face years of repeated surgeries and other failed treatments.

An example of a patient with a more constructive attitude toward his pain was also presented by Sternbach. This patient, Fred, was 53 years old and had been a butcher 20 years ago, lifting, carrying, and chopping 100-lb sides of beef all day. After a laminectomy for a ruptured disk, a staphylococcal infection developed in the incision. Fred was hospitalized for 18 months. He was finally discharged with arachnoiditis, a chronic scarring of the spinal cord. This left him with severe pain in his back and legs. Unable to return to his original work, he used his knowledge of meats to begin a career in the wholesale and brokerage business.

Like Sam, Fred also prefers to stay on his feet in the office. He is a grizzled, tough-talking man who grew up in the Chicago slums. He describes how he hit the bottle after he left the hospital.

"I drank to pass out. It was the only way I could get any sleep. I did that for a year, a fifth of booze every night. Finally I saw what I was doing: feeling sorry for myself. I'd wake up with the same pain I had before, plus a hangover. I quit drinking and joined AA and went into business.

I'll tell you why I'm here. My family doc heard about this place and thought I should come here because you have some new treatments or something. . . . but I don't want to waste your time and mine, so if you can't help my case just tell me, and we'll call it quits. . . . I'm not going to take that much time away from my family, or from my business either."

Sternbach compared and contrasted these two patients: The difference between Sam and Fred is important. Both are brave and tough. But Sam is on his way to becoming a "professional pain patient," disrupting his entire life as he embarks on a career of finding a nonexistent "cure." And Fred is using his toughness to fight invalidism, to keep what is precious to him; and he clearly begrudges every moment away from his usual life.

Accepting the chronic pain means accepting the fact of having pain that is not going to go away. This does not mean that the patient is going to like it, or is giving in to it and becoming an invalid. Rather, it means deciding that nothing more can be done, medically or surgically, to eliminate the pain—and then going on from there.

Setting goals. Once patients have accepted their pain, they need to begin setting goals for their lives. In general, these goals are directed toward work, recreation or hobbies, and social concerns (e.g., family and friends). Goals related to work are extremely important. It never occurs to some patients that if they cannot do their original job, such as nursing or carpentry, they could learn a new one. They always talk in terms of what they were, not what they are at the present time: "I was a nurse, but now I'm retired." "I was a plumber before my back gave out on me." These patients begin to feel useless. They lie around, gain weight, and feel sorry for themselves. All of this exacerbates their original pain problem.

It is essential that these patients be supported in discovering what they can do, not what they cannot do. Those who begin to set goals for themselves in each of the three areas of their lives will ultimately gain mastery of their pain. Those who do not will continue on a downward spiral into invalidism.

Constructive, not destructive, use of anger. Anger often motivates patients with chronic pain into changing their behaviors. Steve, the ex–Green Beret mentioned earlier in this chapter, is an example of someone who used his anger at himself to stop feeling bad for himself and begin night school. Another patient, paralyzed from the waist down and in pain for 8 years after a plane crash put it this way: "I am highly incensed that I must live like this. I don't blame anyone in particular, but I refuse to take the attitude that 'what will be, will be.' I resent this having happened to me, and I refuse to roll over and die." This patient continues to do all the things she used to do—housework, music, and so forth—only more slowly and from her wheelchair.

SUMMARY

Despite the availability of better techniques for the treatment of pain, chronic pain is expected to continue to be a major problem. The role of the nurse is to help patients and their families avoid the development of a chronic pain syndrome. This syndrome, which can be physically, psychologically, and socially destructive, can be prevented through the proper use of analgesics to relieve acute pain and the promotion of healthy coping behaviors in patients whose pain has become chronic.

EXAM QUESTIONS

Chapter 12

Questions 91–95

91. What type of chronic benign pain disorder is caused by violent deformation of nerves by high-velocity missiles?

    a. Causalgia
    b. Postherpetic neuralgia
    c. Trigeminal neuralgia
    d. Peripheral neuropathy

92. Other than the pain itself, what do patients with chronic pain syndrome complain about most often?

    a. Fatigue
    b. Inability to sleep well
    c. Decreased appetite
    d. Nausea and vomiting

93. Which of the following chronic benign pain disorders has no apparent physical signs in 60–78% of cases?

    a. Causalgia
    b. Lower back pain
    c. Postradiation pain
    d. Peripheral neuropathy

94. What is the term used to describe a family member who harms a patient's rehabilitation by continuing to do too much for the patient?

    a. Secondary gainer
    b. Enabler
    c. Malingerer
    d. Antagonist

95. How long after the onset of pain can a patient take opioids on a daily basis before physical dependence on the drugs becomes a matter of concern?

    a. 1 month
    b. 2 weeks
    c. 5 days
    d. 48 hr

CHAPTER 13

PAIN IN THE ELDERLY

CHAPTER OBJECTIVE

After studying this chapter, the reader will be able to describe special pain problems of the elderly, key assessment techniques, and specific approaches used in treatment.

LEARNING OBJECTIVES

After studying this chapter, the reader will be able to

1. State the prevalence of pain in the institutionalized elderly.

2. State and refute a common myth about pain in the older population.

3. Specify a key aspect to be included in the assessment of pain in a cognitively impaired elderly patient.

4. Specify an opioid that should not be used by the elderly.

5. Specify two distraction techniques that are well-suited for use by older patients who are in pain.

INTRODUCTION

The elderly are the fastest growing population in the United States. In 1984, elderly persons (28 million) outnumbered teenagers (27 million) for the first time in history (Harkins, Kwentus, & Price, 1990). It is estimated that the percentage of Americans 65 years or older will be 18% (52 million) by the year 2020 and 22% (65.6 million) by the year 2030 (U.S. Senate Committee on Aging, 1991).

Despite the rapid growth of this age group, education and research on pain management in the elderly are limited. Ferrell and Ferrell (1992a) reviewed leading geriatrics textbooks and found that only 2 of 11 chapters in medical texts and fewer than 18 of a total of 5,000 pages in nursing texts addressed pain management. This is ironic because acute and chronic painful diseases are common in the elderly. In addition, many older persons have more than one medical problem. Besides having the potential for more than one source for pain, they are often at increased risk for drug-drug and drug-disease interactions (Kane, Ouslander, & Abrass, 1989). Special problems, such as pain assessment in the cognitively impaired, still need to be addressed.

Little information is available on how many elderly persons have pain. Most research on the prevalence of pain looks at pain associated with specific diseases rather than pain in specific age groups. However, some estimates indicate that the prevalence may be twofold higher in those more than 60 years old compared with those less than 60 (Crook, Rideout, & Browne, 1984). Among the institutionalized elderly, more than 70% may have pain (Ferrell, Ferrell, & Osterweil, 1990).

Nurses need to be aware of the special s of pain in older patients. This chapter examines common myths about pain in the elderly and discusses the assessment and treatment of pain in this age group.

MYTHS ABOUT PAIN

Some commonly believed pain myths are specific to the elderly population. These are in addition to the general pain myths discussed earlier in this text.

MYTH: Pain Naturally Accompanies Aging

Pain is not a normal part of aging. Its presence requires aggressive assessment, diagnosis, and treatment similar to those used for patients in any age group. Harkins et al. (1990) propose that this misconception is responsible for the lack of research in this area and state that the assumption that pain accompanies aging is no longer acceptable.

The irrationality of this myth is best demonstrated by a 101-year-old participant in a study on aging (Butler & Gastel, 1980). When the man complained of pain in his left leg, his physician suggested that this was normal for someone 101 years old. The man then wondered why his right leg, which was also 101 years old, did not hurt a bit.

This misconception is fed by the fact that although aging does not cause pain in itself, the elderly are at higher risk than younger persons for disorders that result in pain. The most prevalent disorders associated with chronic pain in the elderly are cancer, de-

generative joint disease, rheumatoid arthritis, and vascular disease (Theinhaus, 1989).

MYTH: Pain Perception and Sensitivity Decrease with Age

The myth that the perception of pain and sensitivity to it decrease with age can lead to needless suffering and undertreatment of pain. It can also lead to not treating the underlying cause of the pain.

This misconception has its roots in the assumption that the sensory changes that occur with age (e.g., vision and hearing losses) also lead to changes in pain sensation. The results of research on sensitivity to pain and pain thresholds in different age groups have been contradictory (Harkins, Kwentus, & Price, 1984). To date, no results of longitudinal studies on the perception of pain have been published. Cross-sectional studies have failed to exclude participants with extraneous variables (e.g., those taking analgesics or those who have diabetes or chronic pain) (Ferrell & Ferrell, 1992a).

Muddying the waters are clinical reports of atypical pain in elderly patients who have disorders that normally cause pain (e.g., silent myocardial infarctions and painless peptic ulcer disease) (Clinch, Banerjee, & Ostick, 1984; MacDonald, 1984). Such findings cannot be generalized to other painful conditions in the elderly.

The bottom line is that the evidence is inconclusive whether age acts as an analgesic. In those studies in which the perception of pain was decreased, the cause might have been disease or other factors unrelated to age. Eliminating this misconception could decrease the undertreatment of pain in the elderly.

MYTH: A Patient Who Does Not Complain of Pain Must Not Be in Pain

The myth that lack of pain complaints equals lack of pain is especially true in older persons, who may not report pain for a variety of reasons. A patient who has had chronic pain for a long time may reduce expression of pain. In one study of elderly cancer patients at home, the average duration of pain at the time the study began was 16 months (Ferrell & Ferrell, 1992b). Older patients may think that pain is normal, or they may have many fears associated with the pain. They may be afraid of what the pain means or of diagnostic work-ups. They may underreport their symptoms because of these fears.

Older persons also have a lifetime of experience to draw on and may be using distraction successfully. As discussed in chapter 5, being distracted from the pain does not mean that the pain is absent.

MYTH: Opioids Are Too Dangerous to Use in the Elderly

Elderly persons are more sensitive to the analgesic effects of opioid drugs. The peak concentration of an opioid in the plasma is higher than in younger patients, and the duration of relief is longer. The elderly are also more sensitive to sedation and respiratory depression (AHCPR, 1992). This does not mean that opioids cannot be used in the elderly. It means only that caution is required in giving initial doses and in determining the dose needed for relief. Opioids can be used safely in older patients.

ASSESSMENT OF PAIN

Assessment is the first step in the nursing process in caring for an elderly patient who might be experiencing pain. The presence of pain may indicate underlying disease, and an accurate diagnosis is crucial for appropriate treatment. Assessment is also important for the evaluation step in the nursing process. In this way, the effectiveness of therapy can be evaluated.

Assessment of pain in the elderly can be difficult. These patients often describe pain differently than younger patients do, probably because of physiologi-

cal, psychological, and cultural changes associated with aging (Fordyce, 1978). Cognitive impairment, delirium, and dementia can be major barriers to pain assessment in this age group, and no solution to this problem has been found (AHCPR, 1992). Elderly patients often have more than one medical problem and are taking a combination of medications. Therefore, a thorough history and physical examination are essential. Other factors that influence pain also must be considered, such as physical functioning, psychological state, and the role of the patient's family and significant others in the care of the patient. Because of the complex nature of pain, this assessment must be multidimensional.

The Pain History

As in patients in all age groups, the pain history should include information on the initial onset of the pain and any accompanying signs and symptoms (see Table 4-2). The nurse should establish the vocabulary the patient uses to describe pain. Many older patients do not ordinarily use the word "pain." They may use terms such as "discomfort," "soreness," "aches," "hurt," or "pressure" (McCaffery & Beebe, 1989). The characteristics of the pain should be described by using the patient's own words. This will serve as a comparison for future reference. For the elderly, any sudden changes in the character of pain may indicate deterioration or a new injury and should be carefully assessed (Ferrell & Ferrell, 1992a).

An accurate picture of all medications the patient is taking is necessary. Several different physicians may have prescribed drugs. The patient should be encouraged to bring the bottles along so that the correct name and dose of each drug can be recorded. Patients should be asked if they are taking their medications as prescribed. Often they will stop taking a drug because of a side effect, such as constipation.

Obtaining a pain history may be difficult for several reasons. Patients may have trouble hearing or seeing, which can make it difficult to communicate their pain experience. Asking open-ended questions can help. Patients may "fake" answers rather than lose face and admit that they cannot hear the questions. Another difficulty may be cognitive impairment or dementia. In suspected cases, a screening tool such as the Mini-Mental State Examination (Folstein, Folstein, & McHugh, 1975) can be used. When a patient has problems communicating the pain history, it is crucial to include the patient's family and caregivers as sources of information. They can give information about the patient's pain behaviors, level of functioning, and use of medications. Ferrell and Ferrell (1992a) advise caution in interpreting family members' assessments, however. The information may reflect the way that member copes with the reality of an aging relative.

The possibility of more than one source of pain should be considered. In one study (Ferrell & Ferrell, 1992b), 35% of patients in nursing homes had more than one source of pain; the average was four.

Physical Examination

Because elderly patients tend to be frail, the physical examination should focus on the musculoskeletal and nervous systems. Determination of trigger points and inflammation is important. Trigger points are hyperirritable areas of tissue that may give rise to referred pain when compressed (McCaffery & Beebe, 1989). Motions or positions that may reproduce the pain should be included in the examination. The findings can be valuable both in diagnosing the cause of pain and in determining function.

Functional assessment tools can be included to measure disability and determine the need for supervision and assistance with activities of daily living. Some examples of these tools are the Tinetti Gait Evaluation Tool and the Lawton or the Katz ADL scales (Kane et al., 1989).

Pain Scales

The intensity of the pain can be assessed by using the descriptive, numerical, or visual analogue scales discussed in chapter 4, providing that the patient can communicate. As mentioned earlier, no assessment tools have been developed for use with the cognitively impaired or demented elderly patient. Proof is lacking that behavioral responses (e.g., grimacing, agitation, moaning) are sensitive and specific for pain assessment. Unfortunately, at times, observing the patient's behaviors may be the only method that can be used. This method must be used cautiously, however, because patients in pain often have no outward signs of discomfort (Ferrell & Ferrell, 1992a).

One study of nursing home patients (Ferrell & Ferrell, 1992b) used the Visual Analogue Scale; a verbal scale; and the pain characteristic descriptors in the McGill-Melzack Pain Questionnaire (see Appendix A), which were enlarged to words 3-in. high and listed separately on flip cards, to assess pain. Most of the patients were cognitively impaired, as defined by an average score of 12.1 on the Mini-Mental State Examination (24 is considered normal). As shown in Table 13-1, all but 17–20% of the patients were able to respond to one or more of the scales. The investigators proposed that patients with mild to moderate cognitive impairment can report pain accurately when prompted. They further speculated that the use of such tools is something that patients can learn.

Pain diaries (Figure 13-1) can be used to evaluate the intensity of pain in relation to activities and medications. This type of log can help detect problems, such as specific activities that intensify the pain or a refusal to take an analgesic until pain is severe. It can be especially helpful in older patients, who often may have confounding illnesses or symptoms.

Table 13-1
Pain Scales Responded to by Nursing Home Patients

Pain Scale	% Responded
Visual Analysis Scale (VAS)	44
Verbal scale	65
McGill-Melzack descriptors	80
All scales	32
Unable to repsond to any scale	17–20

Source: Ferrell & Ferrell, 1992b.

TREATMENT OF PAIN

Management of pain in the elderly includes all the approaches used for other age groups. However, a few key points should be considered.

Pharmacological Methods

For the most part, the analgesic drugs used in elderly patients are the same as those used in younger patients. Pharmacokinetic changes associated with aging may require conservative dosing and lead to an increased prevalence of side effects.

Optimal use of analgesics is especially important in the elderly. This includes encouraging the patient to take the medication before the pain is severe and using a time-contingent, rather than a pain-contingent, schedule. When pain is predictable, the analgesics should be administered on a schedule, rather than as needed.

Nonopioid analgesics. The NSAIDs are quite effective and appropriate for a variety of pain complaints in the elderly. Serum levels of the drugs tend to be higher than in younger patients because of a de-crease in albumin binding in the older population. The risk of gastric and renal toxic effects and bleeding is higher. If gastric ulceration is a concern, the analgesic can be administered with misoprostol, or a "platelet-sparing" NSAID could be used (AHCPR, 1992). Some unusual drug reactions, including cognitive impairment, constipation, and headaches, are more common in older patients than in younger ones taking NSAIDs (Roth, 1989).

Because several of these drugs are available over the counter, abuse of nonopioid analgesics is possible (see chapter 7 for more details). Elderly patients with cognitive impairment or memory disorders are especially at risk for this, as they may have forgotten when their last dose was taken. Memory tools for medications, such as daily or hourly pill sorters, can be used to help avoid overdose.

Opioid analgesics. As mentioned earlier, older patients are especially sensitive to the analgesic effects of opioid drugs. Compared with their younger counterparts, they experience more pain relief with equivalent doses. This has been shown in both acute pain and chronic cancer pain. It has been proposed that this is due to altered pharmacokinetics and excretion of these drugs in the older population (Kaiko, Wallenstein, Rogers, Gabinski, & Houde, 1982).

Date/Time	Pain Intensity	Medication/Relief Measure	Activity (e.g., lying, sitting)	Outcome

Figure 13-1. Pain diary. *Source*: Adapted from McCaffery & Beebe, 1989; Ferrell & Ferrell, 1992a.

Ferrell and Ferrell (1992a) recommend special consideration in choosing opioids for use in the elderly. Both pentazocine (Talwin) and meperidine (Demerol) have been associated with mental confusion and psychotic behavior in clinical use with the elderly. Drugs with a long half-life, such as methadone or levorphanol (Levo-Dromoran), should be used cautiously, because they can accumulate in the patient. The reduced metabolism of the elderly increases their risk of delayed toxic effects with these drugs. Appropriate doses of morphine or codeine are the drugs of choice.

Being elderly does not automatically make a patient more susceptible to the development of side effects of opioids. However, elderly patients are more likely to have preexisting conditions that make the side effects more troublesome. Respiratory depression can be dangerous when it occurs in older patients who have chronic obstructive pulmonary disease. Many elderly patients already have problems with constipation, which opioids can worsen. Elderly men may have prostatic hypertrophy, which will make them more susceptible to urinary retention. Managing nausea, a common reaction to opioids, with phenothiazines or antihistamines is especially troublesome in the elderly, because older patients are so sensitive to the anticholinergic side effects, including delirium, bladder and bowel disfunction, and bowel disorders (Ferrell, 1991).

Because of the increased sensitivity to opioids and the increased risk for untoward side effects, doses of opioids should be adjusted for elderly patients. The initial dosage should be 25–50% of that used in younger patients (Harkins et al., 1990). The dose should be titrated cautiously until pain relief is obtained. Pain is an individual experience, and the individual's response to the analgesic is what should ultimately determine the dose.

Nonpharmacological Methods

As discussed previously, physical and behavioral techniques can be quite effective for pain relief, es-

pecially if used concomitantly with pharmacological methods. Use of these interventions in the elderly requires some special considerations.

Skin stimulation. Applications of heat and cold can be quite effective for pain relief. Elderly patients may be reluctant to try cold because they associate it with cold damp weather (McCaffery & Beebe, 1989). It can be helpful to teach the patient that application of cold to a small area does not have the same effect as cold damp weather, and to have the patient bundle up or use a heating pad elsewhere to keep warm during the procedure. Because of sensory changes that occur with age, the elderly may be more at risk for thermal burns during prolonged use of heat or ice. Patients and their families can use timers or other memory devices (e.g., the length of a television show) to keep track of the time for treatments.

Massage and vibration are also valuable relief measures for older patients. They can be taught self-massage, or family members can be taught massage techniques. In addition to providing pain relief, using touch can provide caring communication for a population that may be deprived of touch in their lives. Chemical skin stimulants, such as menthol ointments, are a popular home remedy in the elderly. Teaching the patient that these ointments provide relief by helping to block the pain signal reinforces their use. It is important to discourage using heat concurrently with the chemical stimulants. Doing so can increase the risk of thermal burns and affect the absorption rate of creams that contain medications such as aspirin (Ferrell & Ferrell, 1992b).

Transcutaneous electrical nerve stimulation is effective in several chronic pain conditions in the elderly. These include diabetic neuropathies, shoulder pain or bursitis, and fractured ribs (Thorsteinsson, 1987).

Distraction. Distraction can be a powerful pain reliever in the older population. Both unstructured distraction, such as visiting with family and friends, and more structured techniques are useful.

Listening to music can be especially meaningful to the elderly, as it can evoke pleasant memories. Patients with hearing aids may have difficulty using a headset. If the patient is in a private room, using a tape player should not be a problem. The following case example illustrates the potential power of listening to music:

> Mrs. W. was admitted from a nursing home to a surgical unit with a stage IV pressure sore on her buttocks. The sore involved the sacrum and had fistulas that oozed stool. It was so wide that it took two nurses to do her dressing changes. Although she was given intravenous morphine before the involved changes, Mrs. W. still experienced discomfort, and often cried during the procedures. The staff nurses learned that she had owned a tape player in the nursing home and enjoyed gospel music, but the player and tapes had recently been stolen. When her physician learned of the situation, he donated a tape player. Members of the hospital staff donated several gospel tapes. The nurses played the music during the dressing changes, which helped distract Mrs. W. and promote comfort. Listening to the music did not take all the pain away, but it helped make the situation more tolerable for the patient.

Life review is another distraction technique that works well with the elderly (McCaffery & Beebe, 1989). Patients are encouraged to talk about times in their life that stand out. They should be asked open-ended questions about events in their life.

Pet-assisted therapy is another valuable technique. Some hospitals have implemented programs that allow volunteers and their pets to visit patients. The love and comforting a pet provides can be a powerful distraction. Information about pet-assisted therapy can be obtained from the Delta Society, an international resource center on human-animal interactions, at P. O. Box 1080, Renton, WA 98507-1080; (206) 226-7357.

Relaxation and imagery. Hypnosis, guided imagery, biofeedback, and relaxation can help relieve pain in the elderly. Because of social or cultural preconceptions, they may be reluctant to try these techniques. McCaffery and Beebe (1989) suggest using the terms "peace of mind" or "comfort" rather than relaxation. These techniques may be difficult to implement in a patient who is cognitively impaired or demented, as they usually require higher levels of cognitive function (Ferrell & Ferrell, 1992a).

Education. Teaching elderly patients and their family members cannot be overemphasized. Information on pain and the principles of pain management increases patients' feelings of control and helps them choose appropriate strategies for pain relief. In a study of elderly patients with cancer pain in the home environment, one group was given extensive education, and another group was given the usual home care (Ferrell & Ferrell, 1992b). The education included one-on-one instruction, which was reinforced with audiotapes and written material. The program had three parts: (1) an overview of pain and its effects and use of pain scales and logs; (2) drug management, with an emphasis on the prevalence of addiction and tolerance and management of side effects; and (3) nondrug pain management, including the use of heat and cold, mentholated rubs, massage, and relaxation and imagery. The group of patients who received the extensive education had a significant reduction in pain intensity and severity, a decrease in fears of addiction, improved sleep, and increased knowledge of pain. The findings reinforce the concept that teaching patients is a powerful intervention.

SUMMARY

With the rapid growth of the elderly population, health care providers can no longer ignore the special pain management needs of this age group. Because of common myths about pain in the elderly, pain most likely is undertreated in older patients. It should never be assumed that an older person's pain is due to age. Assessment and treatment of pain should be parts of every elderly patient's care plan. The treatment plan should be chosen in light of the special considerations of pain management in the older population.

EXAM QUESTIONS

Chapter 13

Questions 96–100

96. What is the prevalence of pain in the institutionalized elderly?

    a. 10–20%
    b. 30–40%
    c. 50–60%
    d. More than 70%

97. Which of the following statements about pain in the elderly is correct?

    a. Pain perception and sensitivity decrease with age.
    b. Pain naturally accompanies aging.
    c. Opioids can be used safely in the elderly.
    d. An elderly patient who does not complain of pain is not in pain.

98. Which of the following should be included in the pain assessment of a cognitively impaired elderly patient?

    a. Acute pain monitor
    b. Input from the patient's family and caregivers
    c. Electroencephalogram
    d. Computed tomography

99. Which of the following opioids is generally considered inappropriate for use in elderly patients?

    a. Pentazocine
    b. Codeine
    c. Morphine
    d. Hydromorphone

100. Which of the following distraction techniques is well-suited for use in the elderly?

    a. He-who breathing
    b. Describing a series of pictures
    c. Life review
    d. Sing and tap

GLOSSARY

Acute pain: Pain of short duration, usually self-limiting and lasting less than 6 months. The underlying cause is usually known.

Acupuncture: The piercing of specific body sites with needles to provide pain relief.

Addiction: A pattern of drug use characterized by a continued craving for a drug that is manifested as a compulsive drug-seeking behavior leading to an overwhelming involvement with the use and procurement of the drug. A psychological dependence.

AHCPR: Agency for Health Care Policy and Research. Federal agency established as part of the U.S. Department of Health and Human Services in 1989.

Agonist: Any morphinelike compound that produces bodily effects including pain relief, sedation, constipation, and respiratory depression.

Agonist-antagonist: An opioid compound with an affinity for two or more types of opioid receptors that blocks opioid effects on one receptor type while producing opioid effects on a second receptor type.

Analgesic: A drug that reduces the intensity of pain without causing loss of consciousness.

Analgesic abuse: Regular daily intake of analgesics that results in drug tolerance. Usual doses no longer relieve pain symptoms, and increased doses are necessary for relief. Signs and symptoms of withdrawal occur when the medication is stopped.

Anxiety: A state of apprehensiveness that causes physiological changes associated with stimulation of the sympathetic and parasympathetic nervous systems.

Biofeedback: A technique in which a person is made aware of changes in bodily functions, with the aim of eventually controlling the functions to advantage (autoregulation).

Causalgia: A pain syndrome characteristically associated with rapid, violent deformation of nerves by high-velocity missiles such as bullets. The pain is usually described as severe and burning.

Chronic benign pain: Prolonged pain in which the cause is not a threat to the patient's life. The patient is in pain most of the time.

Chronic pain: Prolonged pain, usually lasting than 6 months or longer.

Chronic periodic pain: Intermittent episodes of pain over months and years. Although periods lasting for days or weeks may be pain-free, the pain eventually returns.

Chronic progressive pain: Prolonged pain that increases in intensity. The underlying cause is usually known and is a threat to the patient's life.

Counterirritant: An agent that is applied to produce irritation at one site so as to decrease perception of pain at the same or another site.

Distraction: Techniques that help patients focus their attention on stimuli other than the pain, placing pain at the periphery of awareness.

Endorphins: Endogenous substances that bind to opiate receptors and act the same as opioids to relieve pain.

Epidural: Situated within the spinal canal, on or outside the dura mater (tough membrane surrounding the spinal cord).

Equianalgesic: Having equal pain-killing effect. Ten milligrams of morphine sulfate given intramuscularly is generally used for opioid analgesic comparisons.

Guided imagery: A method of teaching patients to develop mental images that decrease the intensity of pain or become a pleasant or painless substitute for pain.

Half-life: The length of time it takes for half of the absorbed dose of a drug to be metabolized and eliminated from the body.

Hypnosis: A state of alertness characterized by attentive, receptive, focal concentration with diminished peripheral awareness.

Interpleural: Situated between the membrane surrounding the lungs and the membrane lining the thoracic cavity.

Intrathecal: Within a sheath (e.g., cerebrospinal fluid contained within the dura mater is intrathecal).

Local nerve block: Infiltration of a local anesthetic around a peripheral nerve to produce anesthesia in the area supplied by the nerve.

Migraine: A recurring headache associated with a group of characteristic signs and symptoms, usually repetitive, stereotypical attacks with or without precipitating factors.

Modulation: The step in pain conduction in which a neural pathway in the central nervous system selectively inhibits pain transmission.

Narcotic: Any morphinelike compound that produces bodily effects including pain relief, sedation, constipation, and respiratory depression. Synonymous with opioid.

Neuropathic pain: Pain that arises from a damaged nerve.

Neuralgia: Pain syndrome associated with damage of a peripheral nerve.

Nociception: The process of pain transmission.

Nociceptor: A sensory neuron that sends painful sensations.

NSAID: Nonsteroidal antiinflammatory drug. Any of a group of nonopioid analgesics that reduce inflammation. The therapeutic effect is most likely due to the drugs' ability to block the synthesis of prostaglandin.

Opioid: Any morphinelike compound that produces bodily effects including pain relief, sedation, constipation, and respiratory depression. Synonymous with narcotic.

Pain: Whatever the patient says it is, existing whenever he or she says it does. An unpleasant sensory and emotional experience associated with actual or potential tissue damage or described in terms of such damage.

PCA: Patient-controlled analgesia. Self-administration of an analgesic by a patient. Usually refers to using a programmable pump to self-administer an intravenous opioid.

Peak analgesia: Time after administration when an analgesic provides maximum pain relief.

Perception: The step in pain conduction in which neural messages are converted into subjective experience.

Phantom limb pain: A chronic pain syndrome in which the patient feels pain in a body part that has been amputated.

Physical dependence: A biochemical state caused by long-term use of opioids. Patients experience signs and symptoms of withdrawal when the drug is abruptly discontinued or an opioid antagonist is administered.

Placebo: Any medical treatment or nursing care that produces an effect in a patient. The effect is caused by the placebo's implicit, explicit, or therapeutic intent, not by its specific nature (physical or chemical properties).

Placebo reactor: A patient who responds to a placebo in accordance with its intent.

Potentiator: A drug that supposedly increases the potency of an analgesic without increasing respiratory depression or, presumably, the chance of addiction.

Prolonged pain: Pain that lasts longer than a few weeks and significantly interferes with the patient's quality of life.

Prostaglandins: Pain-inducing substances released in response to tissue injury.

Relative potency: A precise measure of a drug's ability to reduce pain compared with other drugs.

Relaxation techniques: Any of a variety of methods to help decrease anxiety and muscle tension. Examples include imagery, distraction, and progressive muscle relaxation.

TENS: Transcutaneous electrical nerve stimulation. A technique that uses an electronic pulse generator to apply electrical stimulation to the skin.

Therapeutic ceiling: The dosage limit to analgesic potency.

Tolerance: Phenomena of decreased effectiveness of a drug after repeated administration. A larger dose is required to achieve the same amount of analgesia.

Transduction: The step in pain conduction in which noxious stimuli trigger electrical activity in the endings of afferent nerve fibers (nociceptors).

Transmission: The step in pain conduction in which impulses travel from peripheral nerve to spinal cord. Projection neurons then carry the message to the thalamus, and the message is continued to the cortex.

Visual Analogue Scale: A graphic linear tool used to measure pain intensity, with "no pain" and "pain as bad as it could be" as anchors.

BIBLIOGRAPHY

Abu-Saad, H. (1984). Cultural group indicators of pain in children. *Maternal Child Nursing Journal, 13,* 187–196.

Agency for Health Care Policy and Research. (1992). *Acute pain management: Operative or medical procedures and trauma. Clinical practice guideline.* Washington, DC: Dept. of Health and Human Services.

American Pain Society. (1989). *Principles of analgesic use in the treatment of acute pain and chronic cancer pain: A consise guide to medical practice* (2nd ed.). Skokie, IL: Author.

Anand, K. J. S., & Hickey, P. R. (1987). Pain in the fetus and neonate. *The New England Journal of Medicine, 317,* 1321–1329.

Andreoli, T. E. (1990). *Cecil essentials of medicine* (2nd ed., p. 712). Philadelphia: Saunders.

Angell, M. (1982). The quality of mercy [Letter]. *The New England Journal of Medicine, 306(2), 98–99.*

Armitage, K. J., Schneiderman, L. J., & Bass, R. A. (1979). Response of physicians to medical complaints in men and women. *Journal of the American Medical Association, 241*(20), 2186–2187.

Bach, S., Noreng, T. J., & Tjellden, N. U. (1988). Phantom limb pain in amputees during the first 12 months following limb amputation, after preoperative lumbar epidural blockade. *Pain, 33,* 297–301.

Beecher, H. K. (1946). Pain in men wounded in battle. *Annals of Surgery, 124,* 96.

Beecher, H. K. (1959). *Measurement of subjective responses.* New York: Oxford University Press.

Bender, L. H., Weaver, K., & Edwards, K. (1990). Postoperative patient-controlled analgesia in children. *Pediatric Nursing, 16*(6), 549–554.

Benedetti, C. (1987). Intraspinal analgesia: An historical overview. *Acta Anaesthesiologica Scandinavica, 31*(Suppl. 85), 17–24.

Beyer, J. E., & Levin, C. R. (1987). Issues and advances in pain control in children. *Nursing Clinics of North America, 22*(3), 661–674.

Boas, R. A. (1976). Chronic, benign pain. *Pain, 2,* 359.

Bond, R. M. (1984). *Pain: Its nature, analysis and treatment* (2nd ed.). New York: Churchill Livingstone.

Bonica, J. J. (1982). Postoperative pain: Parts 1 and 2. *Contemporary Surgery, 20,* Jan. and Feb.

Bonica, J. J. (1987). Importance of effective pain control. *Acta Anaesthesiologica Scandinavica, 31*(Suppl. 85), 1–16.

Bonica, J. J. (1988). Biology, pathophysiology, and treatment of acute pain. In S. Lipton & J. Miles (Eds.), *Persistent pain* (Vol. 5). London: Academic Press.

Bonica, J. J. (Ed.). (1990). *The management of pain* (2nd ed.). Philadelphia: Lea and Febiger.

Butler, R. N., & Gastel, B. (1980). Care of the aged: Perspectives on pain and discomfort. In L. K. Ng & J. Bonica (Eds.), *Pain, discomfort, and humanitarian care* (pp. 297–311). New York: Elsevier.

Chapman, C. R. (1984). Psychological factors in postoperative pain. In G. Smith & B. G. Covino (Eds.), *Acute pain*. Boston: Butterworths.

Chapman, C. R., & Feather, V. W. (1973). Effects of diazepam on human pain tolerance and sesitivity. *Psychosomatic Medicine, 35,* 330–340.

Clinch, D., Banerjee, A. K., and Ostick, G. (1984). Absence of abdominal pain in elderly patients with peptic ulcer disease. *Age and Ageing, 13,* 120–123.

Cohen, F. L. (1980). Postsurgical pain relief: Patients' status and nurses' medication choices. *Pain, 9,* 265–274.

Cousins, M. J. (1991). Prevention of postoperative pain. In M. R. Bond, J. E. Charlton, & C. J. Woolf (Eds.), *Pain research and clinical management* (Vol. 4). *Proceedings of the VIth World Congress on Pain.* Amsterdam: Elsevier.

Coyle, N., Mauskop, A., Maggard, J., & Foley, K. M. (1986). Continuous subcutaneous infusions of opiates in cancer patients with pain. *Oncology Nursing Forum, 13,* 53–57.

Craig, K. D., Best, H., & Reith, G. (1978). Social determinants of reports of pain in the absence of painful stimulation. *Canadian Journal of Behavioral Science, 6,* 169–177.

Crook, J., Rideout, E., & Browne, G. (1984). The prevelance of pain complaints in a general population. *Pain, 18,* 299–314.

Dalessio, D. J. (1991). Diagnosis and treatment of cranial neuralgias. *Medical Clinics of North America, 75*(3), 605–612.

Davitz, L. L., & Davitz, J. R. (1985). Culture and nurses' inferences of suffering. In L. A. Copp (Ed.), *Perspectives on pain.* New York: Churhill Livingstone.

Debetz, B. (1981). A fresh look at an old phenomenon: Hypnosis. *Journal of the American Medical Women's Association, 36,* 109–111.

de Girolamo, G. (1991). Epidemiology and social costs of low back pain and fibromyalgia. *Clinical Journal of Pain, 7*(Suppl. 1), S1–S7.

Diamond S. (1991). Stategies for migrane management (Review article) *Cleve Clin J Med, May–June; 58*(3) 257–61.

Dichgans, J., & Diener, H.-C. (1988). Clinical manifestations of excessive use of analgesic medication. In H.-C. Diener & M. Wilkinson (Eds.), *Drug-induced headaches.* New York: Springer-Verlag.

Didion, J. (1979). *The white album.* New York: Simon and Schuster.

Donovan, M. I., & Girton, S. E. (1984). *Cancer care nursing* (2nd ed.). Norwalk, CT: Appleton-Century-Crofts.

Dundee, J. W., Love, W. J., & Moore, J. (1963). Alterations in response to somatic pain associated with anesthesia: XV. Further studies with phenothiazine derivatives and similar drugs. *British Journal of Anaesthesia, 35,* 597–609.

Dundee, J. W., & Moore, J. (1961). The myth of phenothiazine potentiation. *Anaesthesia, 1,* 95–96.

Eland, J. M., & Anderson, J. E. (1977). The experience of pain in children. In A. Jacox (Ed.), *Pain: A source book for nurses and other health professionals.* Boston: Little, Brown.

Ferrell, B. A. (1991). Pain management in elderly people. *Journal of the American Geriatric Society, 39,* 64–73.

Ferrell, B. A., Ferrell, B. R., & Osterweil, D. (1990). Pain in the nursing home. *Journal of the American Geriatric Society, 38,* 409–414.

Ferrell, B. R., & Ferrell, B. (1992a). Pain in the elderly. In J. H. Watt-Watson & M. I. Donovan (Eds.), *Pain management: Nursing perspective* (pp. 349–369). St. Louis: Mosby.

Ferrell, B. R., & Ferrell, B. (1992b). *Pain in the elderly: Research update* [audiotape]. American Pain Society 11th Annual Scientific Meeting, #202. Skokie, IL: American Pain Society.

Fields, H. L. (1987). *Pain.* New York: McGraw-Hill.

Foley, K. M. (1985). The treatment of cancer pain. *The New England Journal of Medicine, 313,* 84–95.

Foley, K. M., & Inturrisi, C. E. (1990). Analgesic drug therapy in cancer pain: Principles and practice. *Medical Clinics of North America, 71,* 207–232.

Folstein, M. F., Folstein, S. E., & McHugh, P. R. (1975). Mini-Mental State: A practical method for grading the cognitive state of patients for the clinician. *Journal of Psychiatric Research, 12,* 189–198.

Fordyce, W. E. (1978). Evaluating and managing chronic pain. *Geriatrics, 33,* 59–62.

Freitag, F. G., & Diamond, M. 1991. Emergency treatment of headache. *Medical Clinics of North America, 75*(3), 749–761.

Frymoyer, J. W., & Cats-Baril, W. L. (1991). An overview of the incidences and costs of low back pain. *Orthopedic Clinics of North America, 22*(2), 263–271.

Graffam, S. (1982). Improving pain management through staff education. *PRN Forum, 1*(5), 1, 3.

Graffam, S. (1990). Pain content in the curriculum: A survey. *Nurse Educator, 15*(1), 20–23.

Gaukroger, S. (1991). Paediatric analgesia: Which drug? which dose? *Drugs, 41*(1), 52–59.

Graves, D. A., Foster, T. S., Batenhorst, R. L., Bennett, R. L., & Baumann, T. J. (1983). Patient-controlled analgesia. *Annals of Internal Medicine, 99*(3), 360–366.

Grossman, S. A., Sheidler, V. R., Sweeden, K., Mucenski, J., & Piantadosi, S. (1991). Correlation of patient and caregiver ratings of cancer pain. *Journal of Pain and Symptom Management, 6*(2), 53–57.

Gureno, M. A., & Reisinger, C. L. (1991). Patient controlled analgesia for the young pediatric patient. *Pediatric Nursing, 17*(3), 251–254.

Hall, G. M., Whitwam, J. G., & Morgan, M. (1974). Effect of diazepam on experimentally induced pain thresholds. *British Journal of Anaesthesia, 46,* 50–53.

Halpern, L. M. (1977). *Anxiety and pain in postoperative patients: Considerations in management of acute pain.* New York: HP Publishing.

Harkins, S. W., Kwentus, J., & Price, D. D. (1990). Pain and suffering in the elderly. In J. Bonica (Ed.), *Clinical management of pain* (pp. 552–559). Philadelphia: Lea and Febiger.

Harkins, S. W., Kwentus, J., & Price, D. D. (1984). Pain in the elderly. In C. Benedetti (Ed.), *Advances in pain research and therapy* (Vol. 7, pp. 103–122). New York: Raven.

Harkins, S. W., & Price, D. D. (1993). Are there special needs for pain assessment in the elderly? *APS Bulletin, 3,* 1, 5–6.

Harrison, M., & Cotanch, P. H. (1987). Pain: Advances and issues in critical care. *Nursing Clinics of North America, 22*(3), 691–697.

Haslam, D. R. (1969). Age and the perception of pain. *Psychonomic Science, 15,* 86.

Headache. (1987, December 7). *Newsweek,* pp. 76–79.

Houde, R. W., Wallenstein, S. L., & Rogers, A. (1960). Clinical pharmacology of analgesics: 1. A method of assaying analgesic effect. *Clinical Pharmacology and Therapeutics, 1,* 163–174.

Jaffe, J. H., & Martin, W. R. (1975). Narcotic analgesics and antagonists. In L. S. Goodman & A. Gilman. (Eds.), *The pharmacological basis of therapeutics* (5th ed.). New York: Macmillan.

Janssen Pharmaceutica. (1991). Duragesic: Fentanyl transdermic system [Patient package insert]. Piscataway, NJ: Author.

Jacox, A. K. (Ed.). (1977). *Pain: A source book for nurses and other health professionals.* Boston: Little, Brown.

Jacox, A., Ferrell, B., Heidrich, G., Hester, N., & Miaskowski, C. (1992). A guideline for the nation: Managing acute pain. *American Journal of Nursing, 92*(5), 49–55.

Kaiko R. F., Foley, K. M., Grainski, P. Y., Heindrich, G., Rogers, A. G., Inturrisi, C. E., & Reidenberg, M. M. (1983). Central nervous system excitatory effects of mepeidine in cancer patients. *Annals of Neurology 13,* 180–185.

Kaiko, R. F., Wallenstein, S. L., Rogers, A. G., Gabinski, P. Y., & Houde, R. W. (1982). Narcotics in the elderly. *Medical Clinics of North America, 66*(5), 1079–1089.

Kane, R. L., Ouslander, J. G., & Abrass, I.B. (Eds.). (1989). *Essentials of clinical geriatrics* (2nd ed.). New York: McGraw-Hill.

Kantor, T. G., & Steinberg, F. P. (1976). Studies of tranquilizing agents and meperidine in clinical pain: Hydroxyzine and meprobamate. In J. J. Bonica & D. Albe-Fessard (Eds.), *Advances in pain research and therapy* (Vol A). New York: Raven.

Kavanagh, C. (1983a). A new approach to dressing change in the severely burned child and its effects on burn-related psychopathology. *Heart and Lung, 12,* 612–619.

Kavanagh, C. (1983b). Psychological intevention with the severely burned child: Report of an experimental comparison of two approaches and their effects on psychological sequelae. *Journal of the American Academy of Child Psychiatry, 22,* 145–156.

Keats, A. S., Telford, J., & Kurosu, H. (1961). Potentiation of meperidine by promethazine. *Anaesthesia, 22,* 34–41.

Keller, S. E., Weiss, J. M., Schleifer, S. J., Miller, N. E., & Stein, M. (1981). Suppression of immunity by stress: Effect of a graded series of stressors on lymphocyte stimulation in the rat. *Science, 213,* 1397–1400.

Kudrow, L. (1988). Possible mechanisms and treatment of analgesic-induced chronic headache. In H.-C. Diener & M. Wilkinson (Eds.), *Drug-induced headaches.* New York: Springer-Verlag.

Kudrow, L. (1991). Diagnosis and treatment of cluster headache. *Medical Clinics of North America, 75*(3), 579–591.

Kunkel, R. S. (1991). Diagnosis and treatment of muscle contraction (tension-type) headaches. *Medical Clinics of North America, 75*(3), 595–603.

Lack, S. (1984a). Non-invasive measures. *Clinics in Oncology, 3*(1), 167–180.

Lack, S. (1984b). Total pain. *Clinics in Oncology, 3*(1), 33–44.

Lander, J. (1990). Clinical judgements in pain management. *Pain, 42*(1), 15–22.

Laudenslager, M. L., Ryan, S. M., Drugan, R. C., Hyson, R. L., & Maier, S. F. (1983). Coping and immunosuppression: Inescapable but not escapable shock suppresses lymphocyte proliferation. *Science, 221,* 568–570.

Lawria, S. C., Forbes, D. W., Akhtar, T. M., & Morton, N. S. (1990). Patient-controlled analgesia in children. *Anaesthesia, 45*(12), 1074–1076.

Lewis, J. R. (1980). Evaluation of new analgesics. *Journal of the American Medical Association, 243,* 14.

Liebeskind, J. C. (1991). Pain can kill [Editorial]. *Pain, 44,* 3–4.

Liebeskind, J. C., & Melzack, R. (1987). The International Pain Foundation: Meeting a need for education in pain management. *Pain, 30,* 1–2.

Lipman, A. G. (1980, February). Drug therapy in cancer pain. *Cancer Nursing,* pp. 39–46.

Lipton R. B., & Stewart, W. F. (1993). Migraine in the United States: A review of epidemiology and health care use. *Neurology, 43*(6, Suppl. 3), S6–S10.

MacDonald, J. B. (1984). Presentation of acute myocardial infarction in the elderly. *Age and Ageing, 13,* 196–200.

Marks, M. M., & Sachar, E. J. (1973). Undertreatment of medical inpatients with narcotic analgesics. *Annals of Internal Medicine, 78,* 173–181.

Martenelli, A. M. (1987). Pain and ethnicity. *AORN Journal, 46*(2), 273–281.

McCaffery, M. (1979). *Nursing management of the patient with pain.* Philadelphia: Lippincott.

McCaffery, M. (1982). Pain control in children. In J. S. Henning (Ed.), *The rights of children.* Springfield, IL: Thomas.

McCaffery, M. (1982). Pain in children. *PRN Forum, 1*(5).

McCaffery, M., & Beebe, A. (1989). *Pain: Clinical manual for nursing practice.* St. Louis: Mosby.

McCaffery, M., & Ferrell, B. (1992). Does the gender gap affect your pain-control decisions? *Nursing 1992, 22*(8), 48–51.

McGrath, P. 1., Johnson, G., Goodman, J., & Unruh, A. (1985). CHEOPS: A behavioral scale for rating postoperative pain in children. In H. L. Fields, R. Dubner, F. Cervero (Eds.), *Advances in pain research and therapy* (Vol. 9, pp. 305–402). *Proceedings of the Fourth World Congress on Pain.* New York: Raven.

McQuay, H. J., Carroll, D., & Moore, R. A. (1988). Postoperative orthopaedic pain: The effect of opiate premedication and local anesthetic blocks. *Pain, 33,* 291–295.

McQuire, D. B. (1987). Advances in control of cancer pain. *Nursing Clinics of North America, 22*(3), 677–688.

Melzack, R. (1988). The tragedy of needless pain: A call for social action. In R. Dubner, G. F. Gebhart, & M. R. Bond (Eds.), *Proceedings of the Vth World Congress on Pain* (pp. 1–11). Amsterdam: Elsevier.

Melzack, R., Taenzer, P., Feldman, P., & Kinch, R. A. (1981). Labor is still painful after prepared childbirth training. *Canadian Medical Association Journal, 125,* 357–363.

Melzack, R., & Wall, P. D. (1983). *The challenge of pain.* New York: Basic Books.

Merskey, H. (1979). IASP Subcommittee on Taxonomy: Pain terms: A list with definitions and notes on usage. *Pain, 6,* 249.

Mount, B. M. (1984). Narcotic analgesics. In R. G. Twycross and V. Ventafridda, *The continuing care of terminal cancer patients.* New York: Pergamon Press.

Mountcastle, V. B. (1980). *Medical physiology.* St. Louis: Mosby.

Mowbray, M. J., Gaukroger, P. B. (1990) Long-term paitnet-controlled analgesia in children. *Anesthesia, Nov; 45*(11); 941–3.

Multgren, M. S. (1990). Assessment of postoperative pain in critically ill infants. *Cardiovascular Nursing, 5*(3), 104–112.

Paice, J. (1987). New delivery systems in pain management. *Nursing Clinics of North America, 22,* 715–725.

Paice, J. A. (1991). Unraveling the mystery of pain. *Oncology Nursing Forum, 18,* 843–849.

Peck, C. L. (1986). Psychological factors in acute pain management. In M. J. Cousins & G. D. Phillips (Eds.), *Acute pain management.* New York: Churchill Livingstone.

Richter, I. L., McGrath, P. J., Humphreys, P. J., Goodman, J. T., Firestone, P., & Keene, D. (1986). Cognitive and relaxation treatment of pediatric migraine. *Pain, 25,* 195–203.

Roark, A. C. (1991, December 1). How much painkiller is enough? *Los Angeles Times,* p. 1.

Roth, S. H. (1989). Merits and liabilities of NSAID therapy. *Rheumatic Diseases Clinics of North America, 15,* 479–498.

Sklar, L. S., & Anisman, H. (1979). Stress and coping factors influence tumor growth. *Science, 36,* 513–515 Slack, J., & Faut-Callahan, M. (1991). Pain management. *Nursing Clinics of North America, 26*(2), 463–476.

Skyhoj Olsen, T. 1990. Migraine with and without aura: The same disease due to cerebral vasospasm of different intensity. A hypothesis based on CBF studies during migraine. *Headache, 30*(5), 269–272.

Soliman, M., & Tremblay, N. (1978). Nerve block of the penis for postoperative pain relief in children. *Anesthesia and Analgesia, 57,* 495–498.

Spross, J. A., McGuire, D. B., & Schmitt, R. M. (1990). Oncology Nursing Society position paper on cancer pain. *Oncology Nursing Forum, 17,* 597–614.

Stambaugh, J. E., & Sarajian, C. (1987). Evaluation of hydroxyzine versus meperidine in the relief of chronic pain due to malignancy. In *Pain abstracts* (Vol. 1). Seattle: International Association for the Study of Pain.

Sternbach, R. A. (1987). *Mastering pain.* New York: Putnam.

Talbot, J. D., Marrett, S., Evans, A. C., Meyer, E., Bushnell, M. C., & Duncan, G. H. (1991). Multiple representations of pain in human cerebral cortex. *Science, 251,* 1355–1358.

Thienhaus, O. J. (1989). Pain in the elderly. In K. M. Foley & R. M. Payne (Eds.), *Current therapy of pain* (pp. 82–89). Toronto: B. C. Decker.

Thorsteinsson, G. (1987). Chronic pain: Use of TENS in the elderly. *Geriatrics, 43*(5), 29–47.

Twycross, R. G. (1985). Incidence and assessment of pain in terminal cancer. In R. G. Twycross and V. Ventafridda, *The continuing care of terminal cancer patients.*

Twycross, R. G. (1977). Choice of strong analgesic in terminal cancer: Diamorphine or morphine? *Pain, 3,* 93–104.

Twycross, R. G. (1978). *Principles and practice of pain relief in terminal cancer* [Reprint from Sir Michael Sobell House]. Available from Churchill Hospital, Headington, Oxford OX3 &LJ, United Kingdom.

Twycross, R. G., & Hanks, G. W. (1984). Co-analgesia. *Clinics in Oncology, 3*(1), 153–164.

Twycross, R. G., & Hanks, G. W. (1984). Strong narcotic analgesics. *Clinics in Oncology, 3*(1), 109–133.

U.S. Senate Committee on Aging. (1991). *Aging in America: Trends and projections.* Washington, DC: U.S. Department of Health and Human Services, U.S. Government Printing Office.

Visintainer, M. A., Volpicelli, J. R., & Seligman, M. E. (1982). Tumor rejection in rats after inescapable or escapable shock. *Science, 216,* 437–439.

Wakeman, R. J., & Kaplan, J. Z. (1978). An experimental study of painful burns. *American Journal of Clinical Hypnosis, 21,* 3–12.

Warfield, CA (1985). Intraspinal narcotics. A new method of pain management *AORN J, May; 41*(5): 910-2, 914.

Watt-Watson, J. H., & Donovan, M. I. (1992). *Pain management: Nursing perspective.* St. Louis: Mosby.

Webb, C., Rodgers, B., & Stergios, D. (1987). *Administration of pain medication by children.* Paper presented at the meeting of the Association for the Care of Children's Health, Halifax, Nova Scotia.

Weisman, S. J., & Schechter, N. L. (1991). The management of pain in children. *Pediatrics in Review, 12*(8).

Zeltzer, L. K., Jay, S. M., & Fisher, D. M. (1989). The management of pain associated with pediatric procedures. *Pediatric Clinics of North America, 36,* 941–964.

APPENDIX A

MCGILL-MELZACK PAIN QUESTIONNAIRE

Patient's name: _____

Pain medication(s) _____ Date: _____

_____

_____

PRI: S _____
　　　　　(groups 1-10)　　(groups 11-15)

Diagnosis: _____

Time: _____ a.m./p.m.

Dosage: _____ Time Given: ____ a.m./p.m.

Dosage: _____ Time Given: ____ a.m./p.m.

A _____ E _____ M _____
(group 16)　(groups 17-20)

McGill-Melzack Pain Questionnaire

1
FLICKERING ___
QUIVERING ___
PULSING ___
THROBBING ___
BEATING ___
POUNDING ___

2
JUMPING ___
FLASHING ___
SHOOTING ___

3
PRICKING ___
BORING ___
DRILLING ___
STABBING ___

4
SHARP ___
CUTTING ___
LACERATING ___

5
PINCHING ___
PRESSING ___
GNAWING ___
CRAMPING ___
CRUSHING ___

6
TUGGING ___
PULLING ___
WRENCHING ___

7
HOT ___
BURNING ___
SCALDING ___
SEARING ___

8
TINGLING ___
ITCHY ___
SMARTING ___
STINGING ___

9
DULL ___
SORE ___
HURTING ___
ACHING ___
HEAVY ___

10
TENDER ___
TAUT ___
RASPING ___
SPLITTING ___

11
TIRING ___
EXHAUSTING ___

12
SICKENING ___
SUFFOCATING ___

13
FEARFUL ___
FRIGHTFUL ___
TERRIFYING ___

14
PUNISHING ___
GRUELLING ___
CRUEL ___
VICIOUS ___
KILLING ___

15
WRETCHED ___
BLINDING ___

16
ANNOYING ___
TROUBLESOME ___
MISERABLE ___
INTENSE ___
UNBEARABLE ___

17
SPREADING ___
RADIATING ___
PENETRATING ___
PIERCING ___

18
TIGHT ___
NUMB ___
DRAWING ___
SQUEEZING ___
TEARING ___

19
COOL ___
COLD ___
FREEZING ___

20
NAGGING ___
NAUSEATING ___
AGONIZING ___
DREADFUL ___
TORTURING ___

PPI
1. MILD ___
2. DISCOM-
　 FORTING ___
3. DISTRES
　 SING ___
4. HORRIBLE ___
5. EXCRUCI-
　 ATING ___

Constant ___
Periodic ___
Brief ___

Mark E if pain is external; I if internal, If pain is both external and internal mark EI.

ACCOMPANYING SYMPTOMS

NAUSEA ___
HEADACHE ___
DIZZINESS ___
DROWSINESS ___
CONSTIPATION ___
DIARRHEA ___

COMMENTS:

GOOD
SLEEP ___
FITFUL ___
CAN'T SLEEP ___

COMMENTS:

GOOD
FOOD INTAKE ___
SOME ___
LITTLE ___
NONE ___

COMMENTS:

GOOD
ACTIVITY ___
SOME ___
LITTLE ___
NONE ___

COMMENTS

The McGill-Melzack pain questionnaire was developed by Ronald Melzack, PhD, at McGill University, Montreal.

APPENDIX B

ANALGESICS

[In Alphabetical Order]

ASPIRIN
[Acetylsalicylic Acid]

INDICATIONS: For the treatment of mild to moderate pain; fever control; anti-inflammatory

ROUTES OF ADMINISTRATION: PO and PR

USUAL DOSE RANGE FOR ADULTS: 325 to 650 mg q 4 hrs

DOSAGE SCHEDULE FOR CHILDREN:

Age	Children's tablets	Standard adult tablets
2 to 4	2 (160 mg)	1/2 tablet
4 to 6	3 (240 mg)	3/4 tablet
6 to 9	4 (320 mg)	1 tablet
9 to 11	5 (400 mg)	1-1/4 tablets
11 to 12	6 (480 mg)	1-1/2 tablets

SIGNS OF TOXICITY: Tinnitus, deafness, gastric irritation, dyspepsia, bleeding, nausea and vomiting, and constipation at higher doses.

COMMENTS: Significantly decreases platelet activity, 650 mg ASA can reduce platelet action for as long as 7 days; drink full glass of water or other liquid to speed absorption and decrease gastric irritation; give with food, milk, or antacids (or in a form combined with antacids) to minimize gastric irritation.

PRECAUTIONS:

ASPIRIN SHOULD NOT BE ADMINISTERED TO PATIENTS:
- under 18 years of age with chickenpox or "flu" symptoms*
- in last 3 months of pregnancy **
- with low platelet counts
- on anticoagulants, steroids, or NSAIDs or with clotting disorders
- with history of gastric ulcers
- taking oral hypoglycemics
- patients scheduled for elective surgery

---

* Aspirin has been implicated in the etiology of Reye's syndrome, a rare but frequently fatal disease that affects the CNS and liver.

**According to 1988 statement by FDA, aspirin significantly increases risk of bleeding in women who are in the last trimester and in the newborn.

ASPIRIN COMBINATIONS

BRANDS	ASPIRIN	ANALGESIC	CAFFEINE*	ANTACID
Alka-Seltzer**	324 mg	—	—	1.094 g Na bicarbonate
Anacin	400 mg	—	32.5 mg	—
Arthritis Pain Formula	486 mg	—	—	20 mg aluminumhydroxide + 60 mg magnesium hydroxide
Aspergum***	228 mg per gum tablet			
Bayer, St. Joseph's, other chewable	81 mg per chewable tablet	—	—	
Ascriptin	325 mg	—	—	75 mg magnesium hydroxide + 75 mg dried aluminum hydroxide gel
Bufferin	324 mg	—	—	48.6 mg aluminum glycinate + 97.2 mg magnesium carbonate
Cope	421.2 mg	—	32 mg	25 mg hydroxide + 50 mg aluminum magnesium hydroxide
Ecotrin	325 mg 250 mg	acetaminophen	65 mg	—
Empirin	325 mg	—	—	—
Excedrin	250 mg	250 mg acetaminophen	65 mg	—
Trigesic	230 mg 125 mg	acetaminophen	30 mg caffeine	—
Vanquish	227 mg	acetaminophen 194 mg	33 mg	aluminum hydroxide 25 mg + magnesium hydroxide 50 mg

* Caffeine in one cup of coffee = approximately 130 mg.
** Also contains citric acid 1.0 g.
*** FDA advisory panel on internal analgesics has warned against the use of chewable ASA and ASA-containing gum after any oral surgery, including tonsillectomy.

ACETAMINOPHEN
[Tylenol, Tempra, Datril, Anacin-3, etc.]

INDICATIONS: For mild to moderate pain; antipyretic

EQUIANALGESIC DOSE: 650 mg = 650 mg aspirin

EFFECTS: Analgesic, antipyretic, NOT anti-inflammatory

ROUTES OF ADMINISTRATION: PO and PR

USUAL DOSE RANGE: 325 to 650 mg q 4 hrs

PRECAUTIONS:

OVERDOSE: Acetaminophen overdoses must be treated immediately to prevent severe liver damage. Unfortunately, the victim usually feels well for as long as 2 days after the overdose. As few as 3 Extra-strength Tylenol tablets can be fatal to a child. MUST BE KEPT OUT OF THE REACH OF CHILDREN. In November, 1988 FDA proposed stronger labeling on acetaminophen bottles which would say: "In case of accidental overdose, contact a physician immediately. Prompt medical attention is critical for adults as well as for children even if you do not notice any signs or symptoms."

If given in high doses chronically, may exhaust the liver enzyme system responsible for drug's breakdown; may incapacitate the liver's ability to break down other toxic substances as well.

COMMENTS: Minimal effect on platelet activity; minimal anti-prostaglandin effect; gastrointestinal and renal side effects not seen.

BUTORPHANOL
[Stadol]

INDICATIONS: Relief of moderate to severe pain

EQUIANALGESIC DOSES: Stadol 2 mg IM = morphine 10 mg IM

NARCOTIC TYPE: Mixed agonist-antagonist

ACTION CHARACTERISTICS:

ONSET: rapid; PEAK: 0.5 hrs; DURATION: 2.3 to 3.5 hrs
[Plasma half-life = 2 to 3 hrs]

ROUTES OF ADMINISTRATION: IM

SIDE EFFECTS: Nausea and vomiting; sedation; constipation; respiratory depression

AVAILABLE PREPARATIONS: Solution for injection only

PRECAUTIONS: May precipitate acute withdrawal symptoms in patients physically dependent on agonist narcotic

CHOLINE MAGNESIUM TRISALICYLATE
[Trilisate]

INDICATIONS: For mild to moderate pain

EFFECTS: Analgesic, antipyretic, potent anti-inflammatory

ROUTES OF ADMINISTRATION : PO

USUAL DOSE RANGE: 3000 mg per day; may be given once, twice, or three times daily

PLASMA HALF-LIFE: 9 to 17 hrs.

SIDE EFFECTS: Gastrointestinal effects similar to aspirin; GI disturbance and tinnitus

COMMENTS: Major advantage of this drug is its minimal effect on platelet aggregation

CODEINE

INDICATIONS: For mild to moderate pain relief; antitussive

EQUIANALGESIC DOSE: 32 mg = 650 mg aspirin

TYPE OF NARCOTIC: Agonist

ROUTES OF ADMINISTRATION: PO, IM

DURATION OF EFFECTS: 4 to 6 hrs; [Plasma half-life = 3 hrs]

SIDE EFFECTS: Nausea and vomiting, constipation, mild sedation

COMMENTS: Side effects limit its usefulness. Reaches therapeutic ceiling at 64 mg per dose. Most commonly used in combination with ASA or acetaminophen

FENOPROFEN
[Nalfon]

INDICATIONS: For mild to moderate pain

EFFECTS: Analgesic, antipyretic, potent anti-inflammatory

ROUTES OF ADMINISTRATION: PO

USUAL DOSE RANGE: 200 to 1200 mg

PLASMA HALF-LIFE: 2 to 3 hrs

SIDE EFFECTS: Renal toxicity; GI effects similar to aspirin: abdominal discomfort, dyspepsia, nausea, and constipation; CNS effects less common

COMMENTS: This drug has an anti-prostaglandin action. Should be taken with food

PRECAUTIONS:

- Nalfon should not be given to children under age 14
- Prolongs bleeding time by decreasing platelet aggregation

HYDROMORPHONE
[Dilaudid]

INDICATIONS: Relief of moderate to severe pain

EQUIANALGESIC DOSES:

Dilaudid 7.5 mg PO = morphine 10 mg IM/SC/IV

Dilaudid 1.5 mg IM/IV/SC = morphine 10 mg IM/SC/IV

Dilaudid 7.5 mg PR = morphine 10 mg IM/SC/IV

NARCOTIC TYPE: Agonist

ACTION CHARACTERISTICS:

IM onset = 60 TO 90 minutes; IV onset = 30 to 60 minutes; PEAK= 2 hrs; DURATION: 4-5 hrs IM/SC; 4-6 hrs PO

[Plasma half-life = 2 to 3 hrs]

ROUTES OF ADMINISTRATION: PO, IM, SC, IV, PR

SIDE EFFECTS: Nausea and vomiting; sedation; constipation; respiratory depression

AVAILABLE PREPARATIONS: Tablets; syrup, suppository, solutions for injection (concentrated = 10 mg/ml); and highly concentrated (100 mg/ml) solutions for continuous SC infusions

PRECAUTIONS: Use with caution in patients with bronchial asthma, increased intracranial pressure with hypoventilation, or liver dysfunction; older persons may need lower doses.

IBUPROFEN
[Motrin]

INDICATIONS: For mild to moderate pain

EFFECTS: Analgesic, antipyretic, potent anti-inflammatory

ROUTES OF ADMINISTRATION: PO

USUAL DOSE RANGE: 300 to 600 mg every 4 to 6 hrs

PLASMA HALF-LIFE: 2 hrs

SIDE EFFECTS: Gastrointestinal effects similar to aspirin; tinnitus is a frequent but reversible side effect; transient increase of liver transaminase; chronic therapy requires careful patient monitoring

COMMENTS: This drug has an anti-prostaglandin action. Rapidly absorbed

PRECAUTIONS:

- Prolongs bleeding time by decreasing platelet aggregation

IBUPROFEN
[Over-The-Counter]

INDICATIONS: For mild to moderate pain

EFFECTS: Analgesic, antipyretic, anti-inflammatory

ROUTES OF ADMINISTRATION: PO

USUAL DOSE RANGE: 200 mg tablet every 4-6 hours. Two tablets may be taken at a time, but this greatly increases incidences of side effects.

SIDE EFFECTS: About 1 out of 10 people experience some of the following adverse effects when taking ibuprofen: diarrhea or constipation, dizziness, headache, indigestion, loss of appetite, nausea and/or vomiting, nervousness.

SIGNS OF TOXICITY: Headache (increased incidence in doses above 100 mg) dizziness, confusion, syncope, hallucinations, seizures, fluid retention, edema, abdominal pain, black, tarry stools.

COMMENTS: Ibuprofen was previously available only by prescription. But in 1984 the FDA allowed it to be released for OTC sale in lower dosages. OTC preparations contain only 200 mg. Exerts anti-prostaglandin action.

PRECAUTIONS:

- Ibuprofen probably should not be given to children under age 14
- Decreases platelet aggregation resulting in increased bleeding time

AVAILABLE BRANDS: Doan's Ibuprofen Pills, Haltran, Medipren, Midol 200, Nuprin, Trendar

INDOMETHACIN
[Indocin]

INDICATIONS: For mild to moderate pain

EFFECTS: Analgesic, antipyretic, potent anti-inflammatory

ROUTES OF ADMINISTRATION: PO

USUAL DOSE RANGE: 25 mg twice or three times daily; increase by 25 mg increments weekly to 100-200 mg in divided doses. Daily dose should not exceed this amount.

PLASMA HALF-LIFE: 2 hrs

SIDE EFFECTS: Gastrointestinal disturbances are the most common side effects: nausea and vomiting, loss of appetite, indigestion, or diarrhea are common among patients taking Indocin, but incidence can be reduced by taking the drug after meals. Reducing the dose is also effective.

SIGNS OF TOXICITY: Headache (increased incidence in doses above 100 mg), dizziness, confusion, syncope, hallucinations, seizures, fluid retention, edema, abdominal pain, black, tarry stools

COMMENTS: This drug has anti-prostaglandin action.

PRECAUTIONS:

- Indocin should not be given to children under age 14
- Decreases platelet aggregation resulting in increased bleeding time

LEVORPHANOL
[Levo-Dromoran]

INDICATIONS: Relief of moderate to severe pain

EQUIANALGESIC DOSES:

- Levo-Dromoran PO 4 mg = 10 mg morphine IM
- Levo-Dromoran 2 mg IM/SC/IV = morphine 10 mg IM

NARCOTIC TYPE: Mixed agonist-antagonist

ACTION CHARACTERISTICS:

IM ONSET = unknown; PEAK EFFECT = 2 hrs; DURATION: PO = 4-7; IM/SC = 4-6
[Plasma half-life = 12 to 16 hrs]

ROUTES OF ADMINISTRATION: IM, IV

SIDE EFFECTS: Nausea and vomiting, sedation, constipation, respiratory depression

AVAILABLE PREPARATIONS: Tablets and solution for injection

COMMENTS: Can be used for continuous SC infusion

PRECAUTIONS: Accumulates with repeated doses and may cause excessive sedation and other side effects; requires careful dose titration to avoid overdosing. Careful instruction of the patient and family is necessary when an outpatient is being placed on methadone for pain control.

MEPERIDINE
[Demerol]

INDICATIONS: For relief of moderate to moderately severe pain

EQUIANALGESIC DOSE:

Demerol 50 mg (PO) = 325 mg ASA (PO)

Demerol 300 mg (PO) = 10 mg morphine (IM)

Demerol 75 mg (IM) = 10 mg morphine (IM)

Demerol 75 mg (IV) = 10 mg morphine (IM)

NARCOTIC TYPE: Agonist

CHARACTERISTICS OF NARCOTIC ACTION:

IM ONSET = 30-60 minutes; PO = 60-90; PEAK = 1-1.5 hrs; DURATION= 2 to 3 hrs
[Plasma half-life = 3 to 4 hrs]

SIDE EFFECTS: Nausea and vomiting, constipation, mild sedation

COMMENTS: Poorly absorbed orally, thus analgesic effect of 50 mgs of oral demerol is only equal to two aspirin tablets

PRECAUTIONS: Breakdown product of meperidine is normeperidine, a toxic metabolite. Plasma half-life of normeperidine is 12-16 hours thus it accumulates with prolonged use of meperidine. Accumulation can lead to muscle spasms and convulsions.

METHADONE
[Dolophine]

INDICATIONS: Relief of moderate to severe pain

EQUIANALGESIC DOSES:

Dolophine 10 mg IM/SQ/IV = morphine 10 mg IM/SC/IV

Dolophine 20 mg PO = morphine 10 mg IM/SC/IV

NARCOTIC TYPE: Agonist

ACTION CHARACTERISTICS:

IM ONSET = 30-45 min; PO onset = 30 to 60 min; PEAK = Unknown ; DURATION: 4-5 hrs IM/SC; 4-6 hrs PO

[Plasma half-life = 15 to 30 hrs]

ROUTES OF ADMINISTRATION: PO, IM, SC, IV

SIDE EFFECTS: Nausea and vomiting, sedation, constipation, respiratory depression

AVAILABLE PREPARATIONS: Tablets, syrup, and solution for injection

COMMENTS: Good oral potency; can be used for continuous SC infusion

PRECAUTIONS: Accumulates with repeated doses and may cause excessive sedation and other side effects; requires careful dose titration to avoid overdosing. Careful instruction of the patient and family is necessary when an outpatient is being placed on methadone for pain control.

MORPHINE

INDICATIONS: Relief of moderate to severe pain

EQUIANALGESIC DOSES:

Morphine 60 mg PO = morphine 10 mg IM/SC/IV

Morphine IT (intrathecal) = 1/60 of the 24-hour dose of morphine IM

Morphine ED (epidural) = 1/6 of the 24-hour dose morphine IM

Morphine 60 mg PR = morphine 10 mg IM/SC/IV

NARCOTIC TYPE: Agonist

ACTION CHARACTERISTICS: Regular morphine

ONSET: IM = 30-45 min.; PO = 30-60 min; PEAK = 2 hrs; DURATION: IM/SC = 4-6 hrs; PO = 4-7 hrs [Plasma half-life = 2 to 3.5 hrs]

Sustained-release form [Roxanol; MS Contin]
Duration= 8 to 12 hrs

ROUTES OF ADMINISTRATION: PO, IM, SC, IV, IT, ED, PR

SIDE EFFECTS: Nausea and vomiting, sedation, constipation, respiratory depression

AVAILABLE PREPARATIONS: Tablets (controlled-release and regular); syrup, suppository, solution for injection; preservative-free for use IT/ED and concentrated solutions for continuous SC infusions up to 60 mg/ml

PRECAUTIONS: Use with caution in patients with bronchial asthma, increased intracranial pressure with hypoventilation, or liver dysfunction; older persons may need lower doses.

NALBUPHINE
[Nubain]

INDICATIONS: Relief of moderate to severe pain

EQUIANALGESIC DOSES: Nubain 10 mg IM/IV = morphine 10 mg IM

NARCOTIC TYPE: Mixed agonist-antagonist

ACTION CHARACTERISTICS:

ONSET: 2-3 minutes after IV injection; 15 minutes after IM injection   PEAK: not known; DURATION: 3-6 hrs
[Plasma half-life = 5 hrs]

ROUTES OF ADMINISTRATION: IM, IV

SIDE EFFECTS: Nausea and vomiting, sedation, constipation, respiratory depression

AVAILABLE PREPARATIONS: Solution for injection; no oral form

COMMENTS: Less abuse liability, not a schedule IV drug

PRECAUTIONS: May precipitate acute withdrawal symptoms in patients physically dependent on agonist narcotic.

NAPROXEN
[Naprosyn]

INDICATIONS: For mild to moderate pain

EFFECTS: Analgesic, antipyretic, potent anti-inflammatory

ROUTES OF ADMINISTRATION: PO

USUAL DOSE RANGE: 250 mg BID

PLASMA HALF-LIFE: 12 to 15 hrs

SIDE EFFECTS: Gastrointestinal effects similar to aspirin; tinnitus is a frequent but reversible side effect

COMMENTS: Longer acting than many of the other drugs in this class. Has an anti-prostaglandin action.

PRECAUTIONS:

　　Naprosyn should not be given to children under age 14
　　Prolongs bleeding time by decreasing platelet aggregation

OXYCODONE COMBINATIONS
[Percodan; Percocet]

INDICATIONS: Relief of moderate to severe pain

EQUIANALGESIC DOSES: Percodan or Percocet

NARCOTIC TYPE: Agonist

ROUTES OF ADMINISTRATION: PO

SIDE EFFECTS: Nausea and vomiting, sedation, constipation, respiratory depression

COMPOUNDS CONTAINING OXYCODONE:

Percodan (Oxycodone hydrochloride 4.5 mg + oxycodone terephthalate 0.38 mg + ASA 224 mg + phenacetin 160 mg + caffeine 32 mg)

Percocet-5 (Oxycodone hydrochloride 5 mg + acetaminophen 325 mg)

Percodan-Demi (Oxycodone hydrochloride 2.25 mg + oxycodone terephthalate 0.19 mg + ASA 224 mg + phenacetin 160 mg + caffeine 32 mg)

PRECAUTIONS:

Phenacetin that is included in Percodan and Percocet is nephrotoxic when taken chronically in large doses; phenacetin has been banned in Denmark and Sweden since 1961 because of this toxicity

Schedule II drug; high risk of physical dependence and addiction

OXYMORPHONE
[Numorphan]

INDICATIONS: Relief of moderate to severe pain

EQUIANALGESIC DOSES:

Numorphan 1 mg IM = morphine 10 mg IM

Numorphan 10 mg PR = morphine 10 mg IM/SC/IV

NARCOTIC TYPE: Agonist

ACTION CHARACTERISTICS:

ONSET: unknown; PEAK: 2 hrs; DURATION: 4-6 hrs

[Plasma half-life = 2 to 3 hrs]

ROUTES OF ADMINISTRATION: IM, PR

SIDE EFFECTS: Nausea and vomiting, sedation, constipation, respiratory depression

AVAILABLE PREPARATIONS: Solution for injection and suppositories

PRECAUTIONS: Use with caution in patients with bronchial asthma, increased intracranial pressure with hypoventilation, or liver dysfunction; older persons may need lower doses.

PENTAZOCINE
[Talwin]

INDICATIONS: Relief of mild to moderately severe pain

EQUIANALGESIC DOSES:

Talwin 30 mg PO = 650 mg ASA
Talwin 180 mg PO = 10 mg MS
Talwin 60 mg IM = 10 mg MS

NARCOTIC TYPE: Antagonist

ACTION CHARACTERISTICS:

ONSET = PO= 30-60 minutes; IM = 30-45 minutes; PEAK = 2 hours; DURATION = 3 to 4 hrs
[Plasma half-life = 2 to 3 hrs]

SIDE EFFECTS: Nausea and vomiting, sedation, some respiratory depression

PREPARATIONS AVAILABLE: Talwin tablets; **Talwin NX** contains 0.5 mg Naloxone per tablet to reduce abuse potential; solutions for IM injection (very irritating to the tissues.)

PRECAUTIONS:

- Can cause withdrawal in patients dependent on agonist narcotics
- Talwin abuse is more common than that of morphine
- Schedule IV drug

PHENYLBUTAZONE
[Butazolidin]

INDICATIONS: For mild to moderate pain

EFFECTS: Analgesic, the most potent antiinflammatory

ROUTES OF ADMINISTRATION: PO

USUAL DOSE RANGE: 350 to 600 mg initially; decrease to 100 to 400 per day

PLASMA HALF-LIFE: 40 to 90 hrs

SIDE EFFECTS: More common in elderly persons: gastrointestinal effects, direct renal toxicity, direct hepatic toxicity, thrombocytopenia, and sodium retention. Because of these problems, usually ordered only for 1 to 2 weeks to treat an acute inflammatory response

COMMENTS: This drug has an anti-prostaglandin action

PRECAUTIONS:

- Butazolidin should not be given to children under age 14
- Prolongs bleeding time by decreasing platelet aggregation

PIROXICAM
[Feldene]

INDICATIONS: For mild to moderate pain

EFFECTS: Analgesic, antipyretic, potent anti-inflammatory

ROUTES OF ADMINISTRATION: PO

USUAL DOSE RANGE: 20 mg is as effective as 500 mg of Naprosyn or aspirin. Requires 2.5 to 3.9 gm daily for potent anti-inflammatory effect

PLASMA HALF-LIFE: 30 to 40 hrs

SIDE EFFECTS: Gastrointestinal effects similar to aspirin

COMMENTS: This drug is useful in noncompliant patients since it may be given in one daily dose

PRECAUTIONS:

- Feldene should not be given to children under age 14
- Prolongs bleeding time by decreasing platelet aggregation

PROPOXYPHENE HYDROCHLORIDE
[Darvon]

PROPOXYPHENE NAPSYLATE
[Darvon-N]

INDICATIONS: Analgesia for mild to moderate pain

EQUIANALGESIC DOSES:

Darvon 65 mg. = 650 mg aspirin

Darvon N 100 mg = 650 mg aspirin

NARCOTIC TYPE: Agonist

ROUTES OF ADMINISTRATION: PO

COMPOUNDS CONTAINING DARVON OR DARVON-N:

Darvon Compound (propoxyphene 32 mg + ASA 227 mg + phenacetin 162 mg + caffeine 32 mg)

Darvon Compound 65 (same as above except contains 65 mg instead of 32 mg propoxyphene)

Darvon with ASA (propoxyphene 65 mg + ASA 325 mg)

Darvon-N with ASA (propoxyphene napsylate 100 mg + ASA 325 mg)

Darvocet-N-50 (propoxyphene napsylate 50 mg + acetaminophen 325 mg)

Darvocet-N-100 (propoxyphene napsylate 100 mg + acetaminophen 650 mg)

PRECAUTIONS:

- Same precautions that apply to aspirin

- **Phenacetin** that is included in Darvon Compound is nephrotoxic when taken chronically in large doses; has been banned in Denmark and Sweden since 1961 because of this toxicity

SULINDAC
[Clinoril]

INDICATIONS: For mild to moderate pain

EFFECTS: Analgesic, antipyretic, anti-inflammatory

ROUTES OF ADMINISTRATION: PO

USUAL DOSE RANGE: 150 to 200 mg twice daily; increase by 25 mg increments weekly to 100 to 200 mg in divided doses. Daily dose should not exceed this amount.

PLASMA HALF-LIFE: 13 to 18 hrs

SIDE EFFECTS: Gastrointestinal disturbances are less common than seen with Indocin. Incidence can be reduced by taking the drug with meals.

SIGNS OF TOXICITY: Most frequent side effects are gastrointestinal, including nausea, vomiting, and diarrhea. Headache can be a side effect. Alteration in blood coagulation occurs.

COMMENTS: This drug has anti-prostaglandin action. It is closely related to indocin but only half as potent.

PRECAUTION: Clinoril should not be given to children under age 14

TOLMETIN SODIUM
[Tolectin]

INDICATIONS: For mild to moderate pain

EFFECTS: Analgesic, antipyretic, potent anti-inflammatory

ROUTES OF ADMINISTRATION: PO

USUAL DOSE RANGE: 400 mg three times daily; increase by 25 mg increments weekly to 100 to 200 mg in divided doses. Daily dose should not exceed this amount.

PLASMA HALF-LIFE: 1 to 3 hrs

SIDE EFFECTS: Gastrointestinal effects similar to aspirin. Patients still should take the tablets or capsules with meals. Fewer CNS side effects than Indocin.

COMMENTS: This drug has anti-prostaglandin action. It is rapidly absorbed.

PRECAUTIONS:

- Tolectin should not be given to children under age 14
- Prolongs bleeding time by decreasing platelet aggregation

INDEX

PRETEST ANSWER KEY

1. True (Introduction)
2. False (Chapter 1)
3. True (Chapter 2)
4. True (Chapter 3)
5. False (Chapter 4)
6. False (Chapter 5)
7. True (Chapter 5)
8. True (Chapter 6)
9. False (Chapter 6)
10. True (Chapter 11)